SUPPORTING YOGA
STUDENTS WITH
COMMON INJURIES
AND CONDITIONS

in the same series

Qigong in Yoga Teaching and Practice
Understanding Qi and the Use of Meridian Energy
Joo Teoh
Foreword by Mimi Kuo-Deemer
ISBN 978 1 78775 652 6
eISBN 978 1 78775 653 3

of related interest

Yoga Teaching Handbook
A Practical Guide for Yoga Teachers and Trainees
Edited by Sian O'Neill
ISBN 978 1 84819 355 0
eISBN 978 0 85701 313 2

Chair Yoga
Seated Exercises for Health and Wellbeing
Edeltraud Rohnfeld
Illustrated by Edeltraud Rohnfeld
ISBN 978 1 84819 078 8
eISBN 978 0 85701 056 8

The Complete Yoga Anatomy Colouring Book
Katie Lynch
ISBN 978 1 84819 420 5

The Yoga Teacher Mentor
A Reflective Guide to Holding Spaces, Maintaining Boundaries, and Creating Inclusive Classes
Jess Glenny
Foreword by Norman Blair
ISBN 978 1 78775 126 2
eISBN 978 1 78775 127 9

SUPPORTING YOGA STUDENTS WITH COMMON INJURIES AND CONDITIONS

A Handbook for Teachers and Trainees

Dr. Andrew McGonigle, MBBS

Series Editor: Sian O'Neill

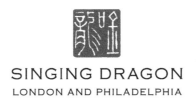

SINGING DRAGON
LONDON AND PHILADELPHIA

First published in Great Britain in 2021 by Singing Dragon,
an imprint of Jessica Kingsley Publishers
An Hachette Company

1

Copyright © Dr. Andrew McGonigle 2021

Asana illustrations throughout the book created by Marie Yagami.
Illustrations on pages 126–128 created by Hank Grebe

Disclaimer: The information contained in this book is not intended to replace
the services of trained medical professionals or to be a substitute for medical
advice. The complementary therapy described in this book may not be suitable for
everyone to follow. You are advised to consult a doctor before embarking on any
complementary therapy programme and on any matters relating to your health, and
in particular on any matters that may require diagnosis or medical attention.

A CIP catalogue record for this title is available from the
British Library and the Library of Congress

ISBN 978 1 78775 469 0
eISBN 978 1 78775 470 6

Printed and bound in the United States by Integrated Books International

Jessica Kingsley Publishers' policy is to use papers that are natural, renewable and recyclable
products and made from wood grown in sustainable forests. The logging and manufacturing
processes are expected to conform to the environmental regulations of the country of origin.

Jessica Kingsley Publishers
Carmelite House
50 Victoria Embankment
London EC4Y 0DZ

www.singingdragon.com

CONTENTS

PART 3: THE UPPER LIMB

PART 4: COMMON MEDICAL CONDITIONS

PREFACE

I have been studying anatomy in some shape or form for over 20 years. This journey began at Newcastle University where I graduated Medical School in 2005 and then worked for a short time as a foundation doctor. Four years later I had completed my first yoga teacher training course and gained a diploma in holistic massage, and I went back into the dissection laboratory to study fascia with Julian Baker. I soon began to teach anatomy and physiology to yoga teachers and trainees. I quickly realized that a common apprehension amongst yoga teachers is how best to teach those yoga students who are injured or have a medical condition, and I started to run workshops that specifically addressed this topic. A big goal of mine has been to make my teaching accessible, fun, practical, relevant and evidence based, and to reinforce my strong belief that the human body is astonishing and robust.

This handbook aims to give you, as a yoga teacher, the knowledge and confidence you need to be able to approach, advise, support and empower yoga students who have common injuries and conditions so that the practice of yoga is truly accessible for everyone. The wonderful asana illustrations that are featured throughout this handbook are of a diverse group of yoga practitioners and it is my hope that through these illustrations everyone reading this handbook will feel represented in some way, regardless of their ethnicity, gender, age or size.

This handbook includes: relevant sections on the anatomy of the human body; an exploration of some of the main injuries and conditions that affect our population; how to adapt certain asanas so that the practice remains accessible for students affected by these injuries and conditions; practices and exercises which can potentially improve or maintain the health of different regions of the body. The material is covered to a depth that I believe is relevant and accessible for general yoga teachers.

I am indebted to the teachers that I have been fortunate enough to have had over the years: Chris Greathead who first taught me meditation back in 2005; Hamish Henry, Paul Dallaghan and Eileen Gauthier who all taught me Ashtanga yoga and inspired me to continue a daily yoga practice; Kristin Campbell who shifted my perspective and encouraged me to step out of my comfort zone; Anna Ashby, Richard Rosen, Sally Kempton and Jivana Heyman who have all broadened my horizons. I would like to give a special thank you to Sian O'Neill for suggesting that I write this handbook in the first place, for being a wonderful editor and for being a constant support throughout the process. Marie Yagami did such a beautiful job creating the asana illustrations and Hank Grebe created some of the wonderful anatomical illustrations that are featured in the handbook. A huge thank you to both of you. Finally, a lot of gratitude goes to my amazing husband Doug who has helped me to remain sane during this process.

INTRODUCTION

Yoga is becoming more and more popular each year. A joint study by *Yoga Journal* and Yoga Alliance (2016) found that the number of American yoga practitioners had increased to over 36 million in 2016, up from 20 million in 2012. The study also found that there had been a huge increase in the number of practitioners who are 50 years old and over, and that three-quarters of practitioners also engage in exercise including running, group sports, weightlifting and cycling. Many healthcare professionals are recognizing the potential benefits of yoga and are referring their clients and patients in order to support injury rehabilitation and/or the management of certain medical conditions. All of these factors result not only in busier yoga classes but also in a much greater likelihood that the students will be presenting to class with pre-existing injuries and/or medical conditions. This puts a greater demand on the yoga teacher and adds to the important challenge of creating an inclusive and accessible space.

What's the difference between an injury and a medical condition?

The term load describes physical stresses acting on the body or on anatomical structures within the body, and these stresses include motion and force. An injury essentially occurs when the load applied to a region of the body exceeds that region's ability to withstand such a load. This leads to deformation of tissues beyond their failure limits, which results in damage of anatomical structures or alteration in their function. This will also involve an inflammatory response by the body to initiate healing. The magnitude of the inflammatory response depends on the severity of the injury and the degree of blood vessel formation in the tissue that is injured (Smith *et al.* 2008).

A medical condition is a broad term that includes all diseases, disorders or non-pathologic conditions that normally receive medical treatment (such as pregnancy or childbirth). The term medical condition generally includes mental illnesses.

The prevalence of yoga-related injuries

There has been a lot of discussion in the media over the past few years about the potential risks associated with practicing yoga, although most of this seems to be based on anecdotal evidence. However, there have been a few studies that have investigated this topic more thoroughly.

In a study by Bueno *et al.* (2018) the authors reported that the injury prevalence of yoga was less than 1% when compared to 38% among soccer players, 19% among runners and 9% among subjects participating in strength training. In a national cross-sectional survey in Germany by Cramer *et al.* (2019) an average of 0.60 injuries per 1000 hours of yoga practice was reported. Based on this, the authors stated that yoga appears to be as safe or safer when compared to other exercise types. They commented that adverse events were more common in participants with a pre-existing medical condition and among participants who did yoga on their own without prior or current supervision by a teacher. In a study by Wiese *et al.* (2019) the authors stated that the number of injuries reported by yoga participants per years of practice exposure was low and the occurrence of serious injuries in yoga was infrequent compared to other physical activities, suggesting that yoga is not a high-risk physical activity. A systematic review and meta-analysis of literature by Cramer *et al.* (2015) suggested that yoga is as safe as other forms of physical activity.

Preventing injury

As we have just discussed, all physical activity brings with it the risk of injury, and yoga is no exception. The practice of ahimsa (non-violence) as part of the yogic philosophy no doubt complicates things here for yoga teachers who can often feel responsible for constantly protecting their students against injury.

There are a couple of practical things that we could do as yoga teachers to reduce the risk of a student getting injured: we could avoid applying force if we are offering 'adjustments' and instead use touch to simply bring awareness to a certain area of the body or as a directional cue; we could offer a student who has osteoporosis the support of a chair or a wall during a balance pose to reduce their risk of falling. Continuing to encourage our students to cultivate body awareness is also significant here. This involves an attentional focus on and awareness of body position (proprioception) and internal body sensations (interoception). By focusing on controlled, breath-led movement that is in a pain-free range we may be able to decrease the incidence of injuries in our classes.

Having said all of this, there are many things that are just out of our control as yoga teachers and yoga practitioners, and injuries will still continue to occur regardless of how cautious we are or how many yoga blankets we wrap ourselves up in.

It is worth noting that sleep has been found to an important factor here. A study by Johnston *et al.* (2019) looking at an endurance sporting population suggested that sleep quantity should be considered to minimize an increased risk of new injuries. The study also highlights a lag period between low sleep quantity and its subsequent impact on new injury risk.

Does flexibility play a role in reducing the risk of sports-related injury?

This is a controversial topic and one that will hopefully become more clearly understood over time. A systematic review by Small, McNaughton and Matthews (2008) concluded that there is moderate to strong evidence that routine application of static stretching does not reduce overall injury rates. They reported that there is preliminary evidence, however, that static stretching may reduce musculotendinous injuries. A review by McHugh and Cosgrave (2010) concluded that the general consensus is that stretching in addition to warm-up does not affect the incidence of overuse injuries. There is evidence that pre-participation stretching reduces the incidence of muscle strains but there is a need for further investigation. A literature review by Ingraham (2003) reported that increasing range of motion beyond function through stretching is not beneficial and can actually cause injury and decrease performance.

The role of alignment

There are many different definitions of alignment in a yoga context. Many teachers and practitioners have the idea that there is one ideal form for each asana and this is considered 'good alignment'. Therefore, any deviation from this form is considered 'bad alignment'. The way you choose to align the different parts of your body in any particular asana will depend on many factors including your intent for practicing that asana, your unique anatomy, whether you are injured or not, what your pain-free range of movement currently is, et cetera. Aligning your knee directly above your ankle and in line with your second toe in Warrior 1 (Virabhadrasana I) does not necessarily prevent you from injuring your knee in this asana. Having your knee in this precise position could cause you to align your ankle joint and hip joint in such a way that the resulting forces on your knee joint are injurious. It is much more important to find a position that feels comfortable for your knee rather than try to fit your body into a predetermined shape. It is all about function over form. In my eyes there is no such thing as universally good or bad alignment. Each asana that is practiced is as unique as the practitioner. There is no 'one size fits all'.

The structure of the handbook

The next chapter focuses on effective and appropriate ways to communicate with students about their current wellbeing. We will discuss why we communicate with our students about this topic and explore some guidelines for going about this.

Each main chapter will then focus on a specific region of the body, starting with the foot and ankle, and ending with the elbow, wrist and hand. Each of these chapters will include the following.

- A relevant review of the anatomy of that region. Topographical anatomy helps us to understand the constituents of our body. However, it is important to note that no anatomical structure functions in isolation, and the mechanical load encountered anywhere in the body is distributed through a continuous network of fascia, ligaments and muscles supporting the entire skeleton. As I am sure you are aware, the human body is extremely complex, and the anatomy sections throughout this book just scratch the surface. I have purposefully kept the information as relevant as possible to the practice of yoga and to yoga teachers.

- An exploration of some of the common injuries and conditions that can affect that particular part of the body. I have included this section simply to allow yoga teachers and practitioners to become a little bit more familiar with these common injuries and conditions. Each person's experience of an injury or condition is entirely unique to them and an individualized approach to each student should always be taken.

- An exploration of some variations of specific asanas so that the practice can remain accessible for students who have a particular injury and/or medical condition.

- A discussion about potential ways to improve or maintain the health of this region of the body. I have chosen this particular topic, rather than looking at the specific topic of injury rehabilitation, which goes beyond the scope of practice for general yoga teachers: not attempting to diagnose, treat or offer medical advice to students. The details here are by no means exhaustive and this section in particular is simply intended to be a guide. The suggestions are not a replacement for the personal advice of a healthcare professional. I have filmed a series of classes for the online platform Movement for Modern Life that incorporate most of the specific practices that are covered in these sections. You will find links to the classes at the beginning of each part: The Lower Limb and Pelvis, The Spine and Trunk, The Upper Limb and Common Medical Conditions.

I have included a brief chapter looking at some of the most common medical conditions and any relevant information about these conditions in relation to yoga.

I have also included a glossary of some of the main anatomical and medical terms that I have used throughout the book. Anatomical and medical language tends to be universal in most cases. The inclusion of this language has helped the writing to flow better. While I personally think that it is best to avoid the use of a lot of anatomical language when we are teaching yoga so as to not alienate or confuse the students, I am hoping that the inclusion of this language in the handbook will help to make it more familiar to you and therefore assist you as you continue on our anatomy and physiology journey.

There is a huge list of all the references that I have included throughout the book in alphabetical order. Those of you who are interested can dive in here to get more information about specific topics.

Finally, there is a further reading section with some great resources for those of you who wish to explore certain topics or subjects in greater depth.

LEVELS OF EVIDENCE

When searching for evidence-based information, one should select the highest level of evidence possible: systematic reviews or meta-analysis. Systematic reviews, meta-analysis and critically appraised topics or articles have all gone through an evaluation process: they have been 'filtered'. Information that has not been critically appraised is considered 'unfiltered'. It is important to recognize that high levels of evidence may not exist for a particular question or topic. If this is the case, you need to move on to the next best level. In writing this handbook I have kept the following levels of evidence (Greenhalgh 2000) in mind:

1. Meta-analysis: a systematic review that uses quantitative methods to summarize the results. Systematic review: an article in which the authors have systematically searched for, appraised and summarized all of the medical literature for a specific topic.

2. Critically appraised topic: authors of critically appraised topics evaluate and synthesize multiple research studies.

3. Critically appraised articles: authors of critically appraised individual articles evaluate and synopsize individual research studies.

4. Randomized controlled trials (RCTs): RCTs include a randomized group of patients in an experimental group and a control group. These groups are followed up for the variables or outcomes of interest.

5. Cohort study: identifies two groups (cohorts) of patients, one which received the exposure of interest, and one which did not, and follows these cohorts forward for the outcome of interest.

6. Case-control study: involves identifying patients who have the outcome of interest (cases) and control patients without the same outcome and looks to see if they had the exposure of interest.

7. Background information and expert opinion: handbooks, encyclopedias and textbooks often provide a good foundation or introduction and often include generalized information about a condition. While background information presents a convenient summary, it takes time for this type of literature to be published and therefore it might not be up to date.

COMMUNICATING WITH STUDENTS

Why do we check in with students at the start of a class?

I personally do not like being called a yoga 'instructor'. My job is not to read a script and tell people what to do or what to feel. I believe that my role is to guide, to offer suggestions and to *teach*. My goal is to facilitate the students during their practice as they turn their attention inwards, so that they can develop deeper awareness and tune into their body-mind-spirit connection. That is after all the essence of yoga. Communicating effectively with the yoga students about their current state of wellbeing helps me to achieve this goal. It gives me the opportunity to offer any relevant advice, suggest alternative options or variations for certain asanas that we will be exploring and provide appropriate props. The communication also invites the students to reflect on how they are feeling and why they have come to practice, and to take their share of the responsibility.

Most of us are not trained yoga therapists or healthcare practitioners. As we discussed in the previous chapter, we are not qualified to diagnose or treat our students. Exploring the topic of why we check in with students about their wellbeing can be a helpful and humbling reminder that we should aim not to rise above our station as yoga teachers. It is important to be honest with ourselves and with our students, and this might mean saying 'I don't know' or 'That goes beyond my skill set' quite often. I have a medical degree, but I am no longer registered as a doctor. I use my background to educate but I draw a clear boundary when it comes to teaching yoga.

Sometimes by checking in with a student it becomes apparent that it is not appropriate for them to take part in the class. They might have sprained their ankle on the way to the class (refer to the box titled 'The PEACE and LOVE approach' below for more details), they might be in their first trimester of pregnancy (some studios that I have taught at will not admit women who are in the first 12 weeks of their pregnancy) or they might have recently had surgery and not yet been given the go-ahead from their healthcare practitioner. I even once had a student who came to a hot yoga class straight from after-work drinks. If it feels appropriate you can point the student in the direction of an experienced Pilates teacher, pre or postnatal yoga teacher, physiotherapist or osteopath. The size of the class that you are teaching is also something to bear in mind: for a student who is newer to yoga you might decide that it is better for them to start off in a smaller group or one-to-one setting. The style of yoga or the level of the class that you are teaching might also need consideration: a level 3 Vinyasa Flow class might not be the most appropriate setting for someone who is working with a painful shoulder but you might be able suggest another, more suitable class that you teach.

Connecting with our students allows us to remind them that while we may be offering suggestions during the class, it is really up to them to make the choices that feel appropriate. It is often important to give them permission to decrease the intensity at any stage or to rest. I often share with students that my definition of an 'advanced' yoga practitioner is one who takes rest when they need it.

THE PEACE AND LOVE APPROACH

Over the years there have been many acronyms to guide the management of soft tissue injuries. Many of you will have come across the RICE acronym (rest, ice, compression and elevation) which focuses on the treatment of acute injury (recent occurrence). Dubois and Esculier (2019) suggested two new acronyms that are based on the latest research regarding tissue healing and cover the acute, sub-acute and chronic stages: PEACE and LOVE.

Immediately after a soft tissue injury, the authors suggest the following guidelines.

- P is for protect. One should restrict movement for one to three days following the occurrence of the injury, which involves not applying load but also minimizing complete rest.

- E is for elevation. Raising the injured area above the heart helps fluid to flow out of injured tissue.

- A is for avoiding anti-inflammatory medication, which may be detrimental for long-term tissue healing. Icing an injury can also potentially delay the healing process.

- C is for compression, to reduce swelling.

- E is for education on the benefits of an active approach to recovery.

After the first days have passed, the authors suggest the following guidelines.

- L is for load. Optimal loading without exacerbating pain.

- O is for optimism. Psychological factors such as catastrophizing, depression and fear can represent barriers to recovery (we will discuss this more later in the book).

- V is for vascularization. Pain-free cardiovascular activity should be started a few days after injury.

- E is for exercise, to help to restore mobility, strength and proprioception early after injury.

Basic guidelines for communication

We will now discuss some of the most appropriate and effective ways to ask a group of students about their current wellbeing.

I suggest that you avoid creating an open forum where students discuss their injuries and conditions with you in front of the whole group. This will discourage the shyer students or those who may have a private matter that they would like to discuss from coming forward. Some teachers like to start the students in a supine position and invite them to raise a hand or place one hand on their abdomen if they have something that they need to discuss. It is a good idea to try to be the first person in the space, when possible. This helps me to begin to set up the space and observe the students as they arrive (which can also help me to see who I might need to speak to in more detail) and allows me to engage with each student as they arrive. As more students arrive, I then address the whole group about five minutes prior to the start of the class to gauge who needs my attention, and then speak to the last few arrivals directly just before the class begins. As you approach a student who is sitting it is always a good idea to come down to their level, introduce yourself if they are new and ask their name. This might seem glaringly obvious, but it is worth taking a moment to consider how important this can be.

We can now explore some ways to phrase the questions that we can ask our students about their wellbeing. General questions such as 'Who has something that they feel they need to share with me?' can open a can of worms and have every hand in the class raising. I had a nightmare once that I asked this question at the start of a class and literally every hand went up. There were stories being shared about a new pet, a recent holiday to Spain and a granddaughter's graduation, and by the time I had spoken to everyone we were halfway through the allotted time. I woke up in a cold sweat. There is no perfect way to enquire. Be willing to adapt the language you use to the specific group that is in front of you and to the environment that you are in. If you keep finding that it only becomes apparent halfway through a class that someone should have spoken to you about their health, you can use this is an opportunity to refine your approach and/or the phrases you are using. One phrase that might help is, 'If you are new to yoga or have something going on that might affect your practice today please let me know.' For an older demographic it might be useful to say, 'Let me know if you have problems getting down onto the floor or getting back up again.' This will quickly give you a lot of relevant information. It is important to note that if you ask specifically about injuries and medical conditions, there will probably be the assumption that you will then understand all of the terminology that you are about to be given. Having said that, there are occasions when it is important to enquire about something specific; for example, if you are planning on teaching Shoulderstand (Salamba Sarvangasana) during the class, you need to ask if anyone has uncontrolled high blood pressure (we will talk more about this in Part 4 'Common Medical Conditions'). It is also important to remember that not all disabilities, illnesses or conditions are visible. With the group that you are teaching you might want to phrase your enquiry in a way that includes mental health. This will help certain students to feel seen and included.

When a student shares with you some weird and wonderful injury or condition it is so easy as the teacher to feel overwhelmed and insecure because we are not a walking medical textbook. Take a breath and feel secure in the knowledge that the scenario can always be approached in a simple, logical way. Instead of getting caught up in all the fancy terminology, simply ask the student how the injury or condition currently affects them. Are there particular movements or positions that feel challenging or painful? For an injury it is useful to know how long ago it happened. If a student sprained their ankle a few days ago then it might be appropriate for them to join the class as long as they practice gently and stay within pain-free range of movement. If they have been working with an injury for months you might decide that they actually need very little guidance and know exactly how to manage themselves. Find out if the student is under the guidance of a healthcare practitioner and that they have been given the go-ahead to practice.

Everyone's experience of an injury or condition is completely unique to them. An individualized approach is absolutely key. Teach the student, not the injury or condition. It is essential to avoid the trap of telling students what their experience is going to be; for example, 'Avoid spinal flexion because it will feel painful.' No amount of experience gives any teacher the ability to predict the future. A more appropriate way of phrasing this would be to say, 'I suggest paying close attention to how your back feels during the different positions and movements that we explore, always backing off if you feel strong discomfort.'

With the information that we have gathered we can now potentially offer the student some helpful advice. Earlier we touched on the importance of giving permission to rest. The chances are there will be particular asanas that you have planned to teach that you need to offer some specific guidance around. This is also a great opportunity to suggest the use of certain props. If you do not have access to props it is a good idea to carry a few with you or be willing to get creative. I have used a spare yoga mat, my sweater and a textbook as props in the past. Do not assume that every student will listen to your carefully curated advice. I feel like my guidance is ignored a lot of the time and my fragile ego gets bruised frequently. We can only do our best and take our share of the responsibility.

The end of the class is a good opportunity to check back in with the students to see how they feel after the practice and if they need any further guidance. This will also encourage them to reflect on their experience.

Here are my key messages when it comes to communicating effectively with students.

- Be open to adapting the way you enquire about a student's wellbeing.

- Do not get intimidated by medical terminology. Find out how an injury or condition affects the student.

- Teach the student and not the injury or condition.

- An individualized approach is key. No two people experience the same injury or condition in exactly the same way.

- Don't try to predict the future.

Part 1

THE LOWER LIMB AND PELVIS

A free online class incorporating most of the practices described in this part can be found at https://lddy.no/pat4.

Chapter 1

THE FOOT AND ANKLE

The anatomy of the foot

*'The human foot is a masterpiece of
engineering and a work of art.'*
LEONARDO DA VINCI[1]

Our feet are a wonderful example of how the human body so often performs very different functions with equal grace. They can support our entire body weight when we are stationary and also serve as a lever to propel us as we perform dynamic movements during walking, running or jumping. It is a blend of short bones, long bones, muscles, tendons, ligaments, fascia, blood vessels and nerve endings that allows the foot to accomplish these distinctive functions. When one really takes a moment to reflect on all of this it is hard not to be in awe of this incredible part of our body.

It is widely recognized that the soles of our feet have more nerve endings than any other part of the body. The heel, the balls of the feet and the toes are especially sensitive since these are the parts that connect with the ground the most and take most of the impact when we move. The feet therefore play a very important role in our balance and providing information to our central nervous system regarding our environment.

There are so many common sayings in everyday life that refer to our

---

1   This quote is often attributed to Leonardo da Vinci although I have been unable to find an exact source for this.

feet: 'To have one's feet firmly planted on the ground', 'To stand on your own two feet', 'Get back on your feet' and 'Put one foot in front of the other.' All of these sayings relate to a sense of being grounded, stable and secure. Our relationship with our feet and lower limbs can have a profound effect on our wellbeing. Moving our attention to our feet and lower limbs can provide much-needed respite from mental rumination.

The bony architecture of the foot

There are 33 different joints inside each foot comprised of an average of 27 bones. Yes, you read that correctly: an *average*. While many anatomy textbooks mention that there are 206 bones in the adult human body what is not always so apparent is that there is a range of possibilities here, mainly due to presence or absence of sesamoid bones, which are small hardened elements that have formed within some tendons where they wrap around bony prominences. (You might also be interested to know that a newborn baby has on average 300 bones. As the child grows ossification of the bones takes place and some fuse together while bones such as the tarsals continue to develop until around five years of age (Hill 2019).)

The hindfoot is made up of two bones called the calcaneus and talus. The calcaneus, more commonly known as the heel bone, is shaped like an irregular cube and is the largest of the bones in the feet. The talus sits on top of the calcaneus and forms part of the ankle joint.

The midfoot is made up of five bones: navicular, cuboid and the three cuneiforms. These seven short bones of the hindfoot and midfoot are collectively called the tarsal bones.

The forefoot is made up of 19 long bones: five metatarsals and 14 phalanges. The metatarsals are numbered, starting with the first metatarsal that joins with the big toe and ending with the fifth metatarsal that joins with the little toe. If you manually move and bend your toes, you will find that the big toe is comprised of two phalanges while the four smaller toes each have three. The big toe helps with our balance and transmits around half of our body weight as we walk, run and jump. The fact that it has only two phalanges means that it is more stable than the other toes and better suited to carrying out these functions. The smaller toes act as a springboard for movement.

We all have a sesamoid bone on the plantar (sole) aspect of the first metatarsal head of each foot while a small percentage of us have additional sesamoid bones present in our feet. Nearly one-fifth of us also have additional bones called 'accessory bones' in our feet and for the vast majority of people the presence of these bones is inconsequential (Cilli and Akçaoğlu 2005).

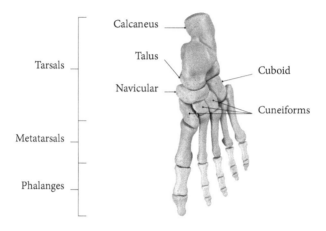

Superior view of the bones of the foot

The arches of the foot

The bones of the foot are configured in such a way that they result in four distinct arches, which include the medial and lateral longitudinal arches as well as the anterior and posterior transverse metatarsal arches (Gray *et al.* 2005). The medial longitudinal arch consists of the calcaneus, the talus, the navicular, the three cuneiform bones and the first three metatarsal bones. The lateral longitudinal arch consists of the calcaneus, the cuboid and the last two metatarsal bones. The transverse arches are found at the level where the metatarsals meet the phalanges and where the tarsals meet the metatarsals. The arches are supported in part by many plantar ligaments.

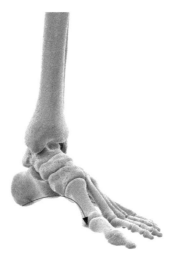

Medial longitudinal arch

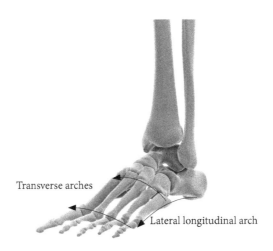

Lateral longitudinal and transverse arches

It has been proposed that these arches coalesce into a functional half dome responsible for flexibly adapting to load changes during dynamic activities (McKenzie 1955). Therefore, when the medial borders of the two feet are placed together, a complete dome is formed. Mid-stance flattening of the medial longitudinal arch when running has been found to both cushion foot impact and store recoverable strain energy in the stretched elastic tissues (Kerry *et al.* 1987). When we are standing stationary our weight is distributed between the head of the first metatarsal bone (essentially the base of the big toe), the head of the fifth metatarsal bone (essentially the base of the little toe) and the calcaneal tuberosity (the back of the heel bone) of each of our feet.

The intrinsic foot muscles have their origins and insertions within the foot. There are four layers of these muscles on the sole of the foot and one layer on the top of the foot. They support the foot in its role as a platform for standing and as a lever for propelling the body during dynamic activities (Gray *et al.* 2005) and play a role in supporting the arches of the feet (Basmajian and Stecko 1963).

The extrinsic foot muscles have their origins in the lower leg and their long tendons cross the ankle joint and attach to foot bones. These muscles move the ankle joint but also play a role in maintaining the arches of the feet (Ridola and Palma 2001). We will explore the extrinsic muscles in more detail in the next section.

Beginning from the calcaneus and extending to the toes is the plantar fascia: a strong thick band of connective tissue that supports and protects the foot. As it travels forward it splits into five sections, each one blending with the tendon sheaths and ligaments of each toe. When the toes are extended, like in our foot position in walking just before we push off the ground, the plantar fascia tenses.

The anatomy of the ankle joint

The tibia (shinbone) and fibula are the two bones that make up the lower leg. The bony prominences at the distal ends of the tibia and fibula are called the medial and lateral malleoli respectively. These form a synovial hinge joint with the talus bone of the foot and for simplicity's sake we are going to refer to this as the *true* ankle joint. The movements of the true ankle joint are those of dorsiflexion and plantar flexion.

Dorsiflexion is moving the top of the foot towards the shinbone. An example of this movement in a yoga practice would be Downward Facing Dog (Adho Mukha Svanasana). The main muscle that dorsiflexes the ankle joint is tibialis anterior. Tibialis anterior travels down the lateral side of the tibia and its tendon then hooks behind the medial malleolus and inserts into the medial arch of the foot (specifically the medial and under surface of the first cuneiform bone, and the base of the first metatarsal bone).

Plantar flexion is moving the top of the foot away from the shinbone. An example of this movement in a yoga practice would be Upward Facing Dog (Urdhva Mukha Svanasana). The main muscles of plantar flexion are gastrocnemius, soleus and tibialis posterior. These muscles are layered, with gastrocnemius being the most superficial, and collectively they are known as the calf muscles. Gastrocnemius originates above the knee joint and is also involved in knee flexion. Soleus originates below the knee joint and steadies the leg upon the foot and prevents the body from falling forward when standing. Both gastrocnemius and soleus join to form the Achilles tendon that connects into the calcaneus and is the thickest and strongest tendon in the body. It is suggested that the Achilles tendon has had an integral role in evolving apes from a herbivorous diet to early humans who started hunting for food over longer distances, resulting in bipedal locomotion (Malvankar and Khan 2011).

The tendon of tibialis posterior passes behind the medial malleolus and inserts into the medial aspect of the sole of the foot (specifically the tuberosity of the navicular bone). Tibialis posterior lies directly below the plantar calcaneonavicular ligament and is therefore an important factor in maintaining the medial longitudinal arch of the foot.

The transverse tarsal joint involves the articulation of the talus, calcaneus and navicular bones and the movements of the joint are those of inversion and eversion.

Inversion is turning the sole of the foot towards the midline. Tibialis anterior and tibialis posterior are the muscles that collectively make this movement happen.

Eversion is moving the sole of the foot away from the midline. Peroneus longus and brevis make this movement happen. They travel down the lateral edge of the fibula, insert into the lateral aspect of the sole of the foot and play important roles in supporting the lateral longitudinal arch of the foot.

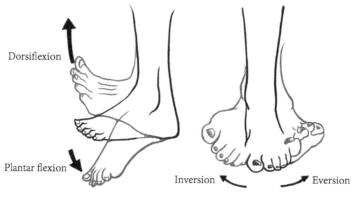

Ankle movements

The ligaments of the ankle joints can be divided into three groups: the lateral ligaments, the deltoid ligament on the medial side and the ligaments of the tibiofibular syndesmosis that join the distal ends of the tibia and fibula.

ARE INVERSION AND EVERSION THE SAME AS SUPINATION AND PRONATION?

Inversion is often used interchangeably with supination, as is eversion with pronation, but they aren't exactly the same. Inversion and eversion are frontal plane motions of the ankle joint, whereas pronation and supination are tri-planar motions of the ankle and the foot. Inversion and eversion are components of supination and pronation. Supination is made up of inversion of the hindfoot, adduction of the forefoot and plantar flexion of the ankle joint. Pronation is made up of eversion of the hindfoot, abduction of the forefoot and dorsiflexion of the ankle joint. Pronation is necessary for force absorption as your foot hits the ground, while supination is necessary for force production as we press off the ground.

THE 'HEART' OF OUR LEGS

The calf muscles can be thought of as the 'heart' of the leg because of their crucial role in our circulatory system. Blood is easily pumped to our lower legs from the heart via large arteries but returning the blood back to the heart is not so easy. Our venous system not only often works against gravity but also does not have the help of smooth muscle contraction in its lining to help push blood back to the heart. Compression of our lower leg veins through contraction and relaxation of our calf muscles helps to pump blood back up our legs against gravity.

The veins have one-way valves that prevent the blood flowing backwards. When we stand still for too long blood begins to pool in our lower legs. Less blood is available to reach our heads and we can start to feel light-headed and dizzy. Our body's clever response is to force us to become horizontal (fainting) so that blood can move from the legs and back towards the upper body.

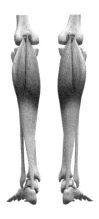

Gastrocnemius

Common foot and ankle injuries and conditions

In this section we will explore some of the most common foot and ankle injuries and conditions that affect our population.

Flatfoot

Flatfoot is commonly defined as loss of the medial longitudinal arch with hindfoot valgus (the hindfoot displaces away from the midline compared to the leg, moving the inner ankle towards the midline). The diagnosis is typically made by physical examination and radiographic findings, and flatfoot can be classified as congenital and acquired, flexible and rigid. The prevalence of flatfoot in the adult population is reported to be approximately 5–14% by different researchers (Bhoir 2014; Ukoha *et al.* 2012; Ganapathy, Sadeesh and Rao 2015). Symptoms include foot and ankle pain and swelling. Flatfoot without symptoms is not an indication for treatment.

The etiology of flatfoot includes congenital causes, hypermobility, neuromuscular disease, rheumatoid arthritis, trauma, Charcot arthropathy (diabetic foot) and posterior tibial tendon dysfunction. Among these, posterior tibial tendon dysfunction (a synonym of adult acquired flatfoot) is the most well-known cause (Lee, Chay and Kim 2016; Sung and Yu 2014). Rao and Joseph (1992) conducted a large study to investigate the influence of footwear on the prevalence of flatfoot in children. They reported that children who wore footwear were three times more likely to have flatfoot than children who did not. People with knee osteoarthritis exhibit a flatfoot posture more commonly than healthy controls, and flat feet have been associated with more frequent knee pain and cartilage damage in people with knee osteoarthritis (Gross *et al.* 2011; Levinger *et al.* 2010).

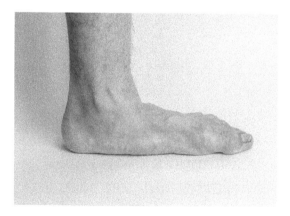

Flatfoot

Plantar fasciopathy

Previously called plantar fasciopathy, this syndrome typically presents with heel or sole of foot pain during the first few steps of walking after periods of rest. Plantar fasciopathy is the most common cause of heel pain, affecting 10% of the US population (Riddle and Schappert 2004).

While the condition is not believed to be inflammatory, the risk factors include limited ankle dorsiflexion, increased body mass index and standing for prolonged periods of time. Dysfunction of the intrinsic muscles has been implicated in plantar fasciopathy (Allen and Gross 2003; Chang, Kent-Braun and Hamill 2012). Plantar fasciopathy is common in runners but can also affect sedentary people. With conservative treatment, 80% of patients with plantar fasciopathy improve within 12 months (Trojian and Tucker 2019).

Bunions (hallux valgus)

This condition involves the lateral deviation of the big toe towards the other toes while the first metatarsal head becomes prominent medially. This condition has been linked to functional disability, including foot pain, impaired gait patterns, poor balance and falls in older adults (Benvenuti *et al.* 1995; Koski *et al.* 1996; Menz and Lord 2001, 2005).

A systematic review of the literature on hallux valgus by Nix, Smith and Vicenzino (2010) stated that:

> No deformity of the forefoot occurs more frequently than hallux valgus. A recent review estimates the global prevalence of hallux valgus at up to 23% in 18- to 65-year-olds and 35% in those over 65, although of course it is difficult to draw a line between normal and pathological positioning of the great toe. There is a higher prevalence in females.

The deformity can often be attributed to ill-fitting shoes, and sometimes there is a familial disposition. It is generally accepted that an imbalance of the extrinsic and intrinsic foot muscles and the ligamentous structures is involved. A link has also been made between flat feet and hallux valgus (Kalen and Brecher 1988). Wong (2007) suggested that narrow-toed shoes may prevent some of the intrinsic muscles of the feet from functioning optimally.

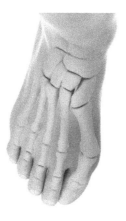

Hallux valgus

Shin splints

Often referred to as medial tibial stress syndrome (MTSS), the term 'shin splints' refers to pain on the posteromedial tibial border during exercise, with pain on palpation of the tibia over a length of at least 5 cm. The incidence of MTSS is reported as being between 4% and 35% in military personnel and athletes (Moen *et al.* 2009).

MTSS can be thought of as a repetitive strain injury (RSI) or overuse injury. A study by Gaeta *et al.* (2006) reported the presence of cortical tibial abnormalities in 100% of their cohort. They also stated that cortical abnormalities can also be seen in some asymptomatic patients.

MTSS has been found to be linked to flatfoot (Bandholm *et al.* 2008) and has a higher prevalence in females (Yates and White 2004). Other intrinsic risk factors are thought to be higher body mass index, greater internal and external ranges of hip motion, and calf girth (Moen *et al.* 2009).

Ligament sprains

A study by Boruta *et al.* (1990) reported that the ankle sprain injury is the most frequently observed injury in the emergency room. It has been suggested that the most common mechanism of injury to the ankle ligaments is inversion of the foot (Balduini and Tetzlaff 1982; Renstrom and Lynch 1999).

The signs and symptoms of an ankle ligament sprain are often weakness, stiffness, pain and swelling with trouble walking or even standing. Generally, these resolve within six weeks but may persist for years (Anandacoomarasamy and Barnsley 2005). The acute phase is usually defined as less than two weeks after the injury (Liow *et al.* 2003).

Achilles tendinopathy

Conditions affecting tendons, which include chronic pain and rupture, are now generally referred to as 'tendinopathies' in preference to terms such as 'tendinitis' (acute inflammation) and 'tendinosis' (essentially chronic inflammation), because this terminology makes no assumptions about the underlying pathology. Although the role of inflammation is still debated, it has long been known that tendinopathies are primarily degenerative conditions and there is usually an absence of inflammatory cells in or around the lesion (Puddu, Ippolito and Postacchini 1976).

The Achilles tendon is one of the longest and strongest tendons in the body, and yet is the most frequently ruptured tendon in the lower limb and accounts for almost 20% of all large tendon injuries (Gillies and Chalmers 1970). Achilles tendinopathy causes pain around the heel that is diagnosed clinically through tendon pain, swelling and impaired function (Maffulli, Wong and Almekinders 2003) and affects a wide variety of the population. The blood supply to the Achilles tendon is age dependent, with the likelihood of decreased blood supply of the tendon with advancing age (Maffulli 1999). The midsection of the Achilles tendon is markedly more hypovascular (deficient in blood vessels) than the rest of the tendon, which corresponds to this region having the highest risk of rupture and surgical complications (Chen *et al.* 2009). More research is still required to more fully understand the multifaceted etiology.

Calf muscle strains

Lower leg muscle injuries are common in both recreational and professional athletes, and they may also occur in middle-aged individuals engaging in nonathletic physical activities such as running to catch a bus or climbing stairs. Calf muscle-tendon unit injuries have been reported to account for up to 30% of injuries in marathon runners (van Middelkoop *et al.* 2007). The term 'tennis leg' refers specifically to injury of the medial gastrocnemius. A long-term study of athletes of all skill levels by Millar (1979) concluded that 16% of cases of calf muscle strain were due to tennis-related activities.

The medial gastrocnemius is more vulnerable to injury compared to the lateral gastrocnemius or the soleus because it is more subject to excessive tensile forces. A few reasons for this are: it has a higher proportion of fast twitch fibers, shorter fascicles and a greater cross-sectional area, is preferentially recruited compared to the lateral belly or the soleus and is a two-joint (polyarticular) muscle (Buchholtz *et al.* 2018).

Musculotendinous strains can be clinically classified as grade one, grade two and grade three based on absent, mild or complete loss of muscle function, respectively.

Peripheral neuropathy

Diabetes mellitus has become one of the largest global healthcare problems of the 21st century and diabetic neuropathy (nerve damage) is the most common complication associated with diabetes (Singh, Kishore and Kaur 2014) with at least half of all diabetic patients developing some form of neuropathy during their lifetime. Over 8% of the general population has peripheral neuropathy, and this number increases to 15% in individuals who are 40 years of age or older (Gregg *et al.* 2004).

Diabetic neuropathy is primarily a disorder of sensory nerves. Sensory symptoms such as pain, tingling, prickling sensations and numbness start in the toes and over time affect the upper limbs in a distribution classically described as a 'stocking and glove' pattern. Only much later in the course of the disease is there evidence of motor nerve dysfunction with distal weakness of the toes, and in extreme cases, the ankles and calves. Diabetic neuropathy can lead to foot ulceration and amputation, gait disturbance, fall-related injury and neuropathic pain.

Varicose veins

Varicose veins are a common manifestation of venous incompetence in the lower limb, and appear as dilated, elongated or tortuous superficial veins. As a result of varicose veins, raised venous pressure in the lower leg can result in skin changes such as hyperpigmentation and induration with eventual ulceration, often referred to clinically as chronic venous insufficiency (CVI).

Approximately one-third of men and women aged 18–64 years have varicose veins (Evans *et al.* 1999). The prevalence of varicose veins increases with age. The evidence to support any association between varicose veins and lifestyle factors such as prolonged standing is lacking.

A study by Kravtsov *et al.* (2016) found that the strengthening of the muscular component of the musculo-venous pump led to the improvement of the clinical course of varicose vein disease.

Deep vein thrombosis

Deep vein thrombosis (DVT) occurs when a blood clot forms in the deep leg veins, particularly in the region of the calf muscles. Pulmonary embolism, a potentially life-threatening complication, is caused by the detachment of a clot that travels to the lungs.

Nonspecific signs of a DVT may include pain, swelling, redness, warmness and engorged superficial veins.

DVT is predominantly a disease of the elderly with an incidence that rises markedly with age (Silverstein *et al.* 1998). Pregnancy has been shown to be a risk factor (Bates and Ginsberg 2001) and the approximate risk for DVT following general surgery procedures is 15–40%. African American patients are the highest risk group for first-time DVT while Hispanic patients' risk is about half that of Caucasians (Keenan and White 2007). Prolonged immobilization, including being on a long-haul flight, is also a risk factor (Gavish and Brenner 2011). When we are on a long flight, we are recommended to do some simple leg exercises to help prevent pooling of blood in our lower legs and therefore the formation of a clot.

Yoga students with undiagnosed leg swelling should be encouraged to seek medical attention before practicing yoga.

Muscle cramps

Exercise-associated muscle cramps are painful, spasmodic and involuntary contractions of skeletal muscle that occur during or immediately after exercise.

Recent literature seems to focus on two potential mechanisms: the dehydration or electrolyte depletion mechanism, and the neuromuscular mechanism. Literature analysis by Giuriato *et al.* (2018) and Qiu and Kang (2017) indicated that the neuromuscular hypothesis may prevail over the initial hypothesis of dehydration as the trigger event of muscle cramps, with overload and fatigue playing key roles.

Stretching has been found to be the most effective treatment in relieving acute fatigue-induced muscular cramping (Schwellnus, Derman and Noakes 1997).

INTELLIGENT MOVEMENT PRINCIPLE – THERE IS NO SUCH THING AS UNIVERSALLY GOOD OR BAD ALIGNMENT

Alignment is a frequently used term that can be used to describe the precise way in which the body 'should' be positioned in each asana. Teachers use alignment cues with two main intentions: to encourage the student to obtain the maximum benefit from the asana and to avoid injury.

Precise alignment cues about feet placement are really common in yoga, from 'Step your feet hip-distance wide', 'Turn your back foot in 45°' to 'Make sure your feet are parallel'. At the start of this chapter we discussed how 27 is the average number of bones in the foot. We each have different sizes and shapes of feet and our right foot is never identical to our left foot. It's not uncommon to have a different shoe size for each foot. With all of that in mind, the more precise a cue is the less inclusive it is. By using precision, we are ignoring the fact that everyone is unique. In the next chapter we will explore the Q-angle in our legs and look at not only how this will impact how we stand but also whether our knees will track over our ankles or not in certain poses.

I used to be incredibly precise with my cues when I taught yoga classes. In Mountain Pose, in order to find a stance with the feet 'hip-distance wide' I'd ask the students to line the mid-point of their ankles directly below the bony parts at the front of their pelvis (anterior superior iliac spines). I'd then ask them to line the base of their second toes up with the mid-point of their ankles to get their feet parallel. In hindsight that might have worked well for a couple of students in a busy class, but it won't have worked so well for all the other students. When it comes to standing in Mountain Pose I now always go back to 'the why informs the how'. When I become clear about *why* I am teaching this pose I can become clear on *how* to teach it. I often suggest that my students explore finding a standing position that allows them to feel tall, engaged, connected to their breath, centered, et cetera. One teacher told me that she asks her students to jump and see how the position they land in feels for them. I love that!

Alignment can be useful as a template or framework, but we must be open to deviating from it in order to make yoga inclusive to each unique body. It is much more effective to focus on what a position feels like and not what it looks like.

Key yoga asanas and how to adapt them

We will now explore some asanas that may present a challenge to students who are affected by the common injuries or conditions that we have discussed above and look at some of the ways that these can be adapted in order to make them more accessible.

Balance poses

While balance poses can have a very positive impact on the health of our feet and ankles, they can prove challenging for students who have existing injuries and/or conditions.

One of the most common balance poses in yoga is Tree Pose (Vriksasana). A helpful suggestion here can be to practice this asana with the lifted foot against the ankle and the tips of the toes connected to the ground instead of taking the foot higher up the standing leg. Placing the hands on the hips keeps the center of gravity lower and this will be a big help too. A wall, pillar or chair could also be used for support here.

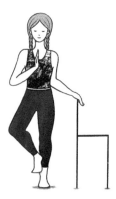

Tree Pose

Dancer Pose (Natarajasana) is a challenging asana that can be made much more accessible by using a strap to bind the raised foot as it lifts behind you. Using the support of a chair or wall in front of you or beside you can also be a great help. Some students find it much easier to balance when they step off their mat for a moment and make direct contact with the floor.

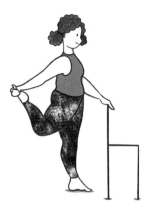

Dancer Pose

The wall or chair can be a wonderful aid for Warrior 3 (Virabhadrasana III) where different distances and therefore different depths can be easily played with. The wall and chair can also be combined so that the lifted foot presses into the wall while the hands reach forward and rest on the back of the chair.

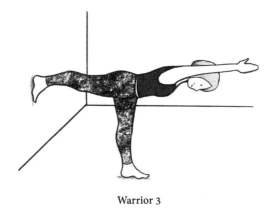

Warrior 3

Poses that require plantar flexion of the ankle

Upward Facing Dog (Urdhva Mukha Svanasana) is a very common yoga pose that is part of a Sun Salutation. For those students with limited ankle plantar flexion, placing the hands on yoga blocks and either keeping the toes tucked under or positioning a rolled-up blanket in front of the ankles will make this pose more accessible. Upward Facing Dog can also be practiced using a chair.

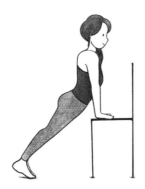

Upward Facing Dog

While Child's Pose (Balasana) can feel restful for some yoga practitioners, if they are struggling with ankle mobility this pose can create quite the challenge. Placing a rolled-up blanket between the front of the ankle and the mat can add some well-needed support here, as can placing a bolster between the thighs to keep the pelvis raised slightly. Some alternative positions include kneeling with your toes tucked under, lowering to your forearms and resting your head on your arms or on a bolster, or Supine Child's Pose (on your back). If the purpose of this pose is to allow for a moment of rest and integration, then any position that feels restful is a great option.

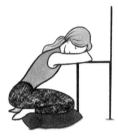

Child's Pose

Poses that require dorsiflexion of the ankle

Downward Facing Dog (Adho Mukha Svanasana) is one of the most recognized yoga asanas. For students with limited dorsiflexion of the ankle placing a yoga block under each heel is a great way to create a greater sense of foundation and support. Placing wide yoga blocks under the hands or using the support of a chair in front will also reduce the degree of dorsiflexion required.

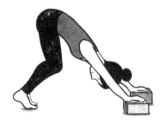

Downward Facing Dog

Garland Pose (Malasana) can look so easy for some and feel almost impossible for others. This can often be due to the range of dorsiflexion available to a student. Again, placing blocks under the heels can help a lot of students here or you can sit on a stack of wide yoga blocks to raise your seat. Goddess Pose (Utkata Konasana) can be a more accessible alternative here.

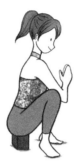

Garland Pose

Poses that require eversion or inversion of the ankle

Practicing Pigeon Pose (Eka Pada Rajakapotasana) can prove particularly challenging for students with a foot or ankle condition or injury. One helpful option here is to place a bolster horizontally under the front leg so that the front foot bears less weight and is free to move a little more. If in doubt, Supine Pigeon Pose is a great alternative here with very similar benefits to be had and much less pressure put on the front knee and ankle.

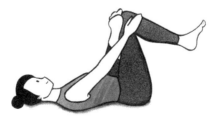

Supine Pigeon Pose

Easy Pose (Sukhasana) does not live up to its name for most of us. Sitting cross-legged can be a huge challenge for many of us, particularly if our feet and ankles are not feeling in good health. Sitting up on blocks, blankets or a bolster is essential here and it can feel really supportive to place a rolled-up blanket between the outer ankles and the mat. If in doubt, finding any comfortable sitting option will work just fine.

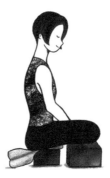

Easy Pose

In asanas such as Wide Leg Forward Fold (Prasarita Padottanasana) and Extended Triangle Pose (Utthita Trikonasana) it is common for students to allow their medial longitudinal arches to fall and as a result the foundation of the pose becomes unstable. Taking a narrower stance can make it easier to engage the feet and ankles and placing the supporting hand(s) onto yoga blocks or a chair takes some pressure out of the feet.

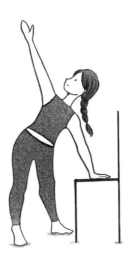

Extended Triangle Pose

Improving the overall health of the foot and ankle

This section addresses some effective ways in which we can all improve and maintain the health and functioning of our feet and ankles. It is intended to be a general guide for yoga practitioners and teachers and is not a replacement for the personal advice of a health professional.

Toe mobility exercises

Learning to lift and spread all ten toes is an important first step towards foot and ankle health. Manually spreading our toes and wearing toe spreaders can also be a welcome respite from prolonged use of footwear. We can then build up to moving our toes in isolation.

This is a good exercise to start with.

1. Focus on one foot.

2. Lift all five of your toes.

3. Keep the four smaller toes lifted as you attempt to lower only the big toe.

4. Then keep the three middle toes lifted as you attempt to also lower the little toe.

5. Repeat this with your other foot and notice which side is more challenging.

This exercise can take a lot of practice and patience, but our toes can become very dexterous if we are willing to put the time and effort in. In addition to this, toe-spreading exercises have been recommended for patients with mild to moderate hallux valgus (Kim *et al.* 2015).

Toe-lifting exercises

The next progression is to sit with your legs stretched in front of you and cross your ankles. Can you spread your toes and begin to interlace them just like you can with your fingers?

A resistance band is a handy tool to have to build strength in your feet.

1. Lay a band out in front of you lengthways.

2. Place the heel of your foot on the end closest to you.

3. Lift and spread your toes and begin to claw the length of the band back towards you.

4. Then give the sole of your foot a gentle stretch by tucking your toes under.

5. Repeat the exercise using your other foot.

6. You can progress to using a band that has greater resistance.

Passive toe and ankle mobilization as well as massage can also be great ways to improve circulation and stiffness in your feet and ankles.

Short foot exercise

The 'short foot exercise' or 'foot doming' is a means to isolate contraction of the plantar (sole) intrinsic muscles. Again, this exercise requires practice and patience.

1. Start in a neutral foot position with the calcaneus and the metatarsal heads on the ground.

2. Your toes need to be neither flexed nor extended.

3. The foot is then 'shortened' by using the intrinsic muscles to pull the first metatarsophalangeal joint towards the calcaneus as the medial longitudinal arch is elevated.

4. This exercise can be performed in progression from sitting, to standing on two feet and finally to standing on one foot.

Lynn, Padilla and Tsang (2012) suggested that training of the intrinsic musculature of the foot should include both short foot exercises and complex single-limb balance tasks to ensure the best results.

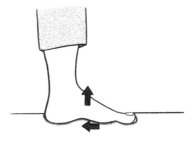

Short foot exercise

Balance exercises

Good balance is an essential skill for everyday life that requires the complex integration of sensory information regarding the position of the body relative to the surroundings and the ability to generate appropriate motor responses to control body movement. Balance calls upon contributions from the inner ear, eyes, muscles, joints and the brain. Yoga offers many great opportunities for us to improve our balance. Shifting our gaze and building up to closing our eyes adds to the challenge. Off the mat, working on single leg raises and single leg squats are effective ways to improve balance.

Ankle mobility exercises

Exercises that focus on plantar flexion, dorsiflexion, inversion and eversion are key to improving the health of the ankle joint. These need to be introduced in a step-by-step progression.

1. Start on your back on your yoga mat with your knees bent and your ankles roughly under your knees.

2. Begin to slowly and smoothly lift just your right heel up off the mat.

3. Then lower your heel back down with just as much control.

4. Notice if you are tensing other parts of your body as you make these movements happen.

5. Repeat this a few times and then move to the left side.

6. Now start to draw the top of your right foot back towards your right shin as you keep the right heel on the mat.

7. Lower this back down slowly and smoothly.

8. After a couple of rounds repeat this with the left foot.

Now we will focus on inversion and eversion of the ankle.

1. Place a foam block between your knees.

2. Begin to press into the big toe edge of your right foot as you lift the little toe edge off the mat.

3. Slowly lower the little toe edge back down and repeat this a few times.

4. Repeat this exercise with the left foot.

5. Then moving back to the right foot press down into the little toe edge and lift the big toe edge up.

6. After a few rounds of this repeat with the left foot.

7. Now try to repeat these exercises without the block between your knees and without letting your knees move.

When you are ready to increase the intensity of the exercises, resistance bands can then be used.

1. Staying on your back, bend your right knee and wrap a band over the sole of your right foot.

2. Straighten your leg (it does not have to be vertical) and press into the big toe edge of your foot, against the resistance of the band.

3. Then press into the little toe edge against the resistance.

4. Now use the band as resistance against you pointing your foot.

5. For resisted dorsiflexion, tie the ends of the resistance band together and loop it under a table leg.

6. Come to a seated position with your legs stretched out in front of you.

7. Then loop the band over the front of your foot and try to pull your foot back towards your shin against the resistance.

Heel raises are a very effective way to build further strength in the calf muscles. These can be practiced seated with the option to have your upper body resting on your thighs or practiced standing with the option to progress to single leg raises. Heel raises with the toes extended (place a rolled-up towel underneath your toes) have been found to be beneficial for plantar fasciopathy (Rathleff *et al.* 2015).

Foot orthoses

Foot orthoses (or orthotics) can limit the extent to which the medial longitudinal arch naturally lowers during normal gait. This in turn can limit the amount of movement available in the ankle joint, which will very likely also have an impact further up the kinetic chain. While temporary support from an orthotic may be needed during the acute phase of an injury, it should be replaced as soon as possible with a strengthening regime just as would be carried out for any other part of the body. Results from a study by Jung, Koh and Kwon (2011) demonstrated that foot orthoses combined with short-foot exercises are more effective in improving flat feet than foot orthoses alone.

Barefoot

An advantage of being completely barefoot is the increase in sensory input received from the plantar surface of the foot. Sensory input has long been recognized for its importance in postural stability and dynamic gait patterns (Kavounoudias, Roll and Roll 2001). Studies like these highlight the potential importance of sensory input to the function of the foot. Barefoot activities, in safe environments, should assist in improving foot function. However, it should be noted that individuals without normal sensation should avoid barefoot activities. Back in 1987 Robbins and Hanna suggested that modern running shoes contributed to high injury rates because they blocked sensory feedback from contact with ground. They stated that barefoot populations report fewer injuries.

Grounding

Grounding or earthing refers to making contact with the Earth's surface with the hands or feet, and a study by Oschman, Chevalier and Brown (2015) reported that these practices have a positive impact on inflammation.

Knee and hip strengthening

Strengthening all of the knee and hip musculature is also important when looking to improve the health of the feet and ankles since everything in the body is intimately connected. We will explore this topic in more detail in the following chapters.

Chapter 2

THE KNEE

The anatomy of the knee joint

The knee joint is the largest joint in the body in terms of the articulating surface area. The position of the knee between the two longest lever arms of the body, the femur and tibia, and its role in weight-bearing renders it susceptible to injuries. This complex joint is comprised of an intricate blend of muscles, tendons, ligaments, menisci, bursae and hyaline cartilage.

The bony architecture of the knee joint

The knee joint is the articulation between the rounded ends (condyles) of the femur and the rounded ends of the tibia. The fibula is not directly involved in the knee joint but is an important attachment point for some of the structures that we will discuss. Hyaline cartilage is a thick and highly organized tissue that lines the articulating ends of the tibia and femur. It serves as a load-bearing elastic material that is responsible for the frictionless movement of the surfaces of articulating joints and is therefore crucial for efficient functioning of the joint.

The patella, commonly referred to as the kneecap, is the largest sesamoid bone in the body and is held within the patellar ligament, a continuation of the quadriceps tendon. The patella is an integral articulating component of the extensor mechanism of the knee joint in addition to guiding the forces of quadriceps femoris to the patellar ligament, protecting deeper knee joint anatomy, protecting the quadriceps tendon from frictional forces, increasing the compressive forces to which the extensor mechanisms can be subjected and providing stability to the knee joint (Fox, Wanivenhaus and Rodeo 2012). The articulation between the patella and the femur is referred to as the patellofemoral joint.

The fabella ('little bean' in Latin) is a sesamoid bone located in the knee joint behind the lateral femoral condyle, embedded in the tendon of the lateral head of the gastrocnemius muscle. Fabella prevalence ranges from 3% to 87% (Silva *et al.* 2010; Zeng *et al.* 2012), making it a normal variant in human anatomy.

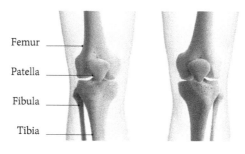

Femur

Patella

Fibula

Tibia

Knee joint

The main knee movements and key musculature

The knee can be thought of as a gliding hinge joint that can roll, glide and rotate. The joint is able to move in three different planes and this offers a 'six degrees of freedom' range of motion, including the primary movements of flexion and extension in the sagittal plane, a small amount of internal and external rotation in the transverse plane and varus (lateral) and valgus (medial) stress in the frontal plane. Translational movement is possible in anterior–posterior and medial–lateral direction as well as by compression and distraction of the knee joint.

The main knee extensors are the quadriceps femoris group consisting of rectus femoris, vastus lateralis, vastus medialis and vastus intermedius which lies deep to the other muscles. Rectus femoris originates at the pelvis and therefore crosses the hip joint as well as the knee joint. The three vasti muscles originate on the femur and only cross the knee joint. All four muscles converge to form the quadriceps tendon. There is a 'screw-home' mechanism involving lateral rotation that occurs at full extension of the knee to create stability. This is often referred to as 'locking the knee'.

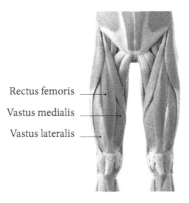

Quadriceps

The main knee flexors are the hamstring group consisting of biceps femoris, semitendinosus and semimembranosus. They all originate at the ischial tuberosity (sit bone) of the pelvis and therefore cross the hip joint as well as the knee joint. Popliteus is a muscle involved in the commencement of flexion of the knee; by its contraction the leg is rotated and the knee joint is unlocked. Popliteus is a major stabilizer of the posterolateral knee. Medial rotation occurs at the end of the knee flexion, again to create stability.

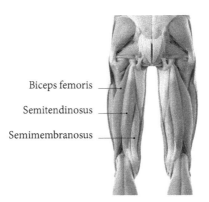

Hamstrings

The knee is laterally rotated by the biceps femoris and medially rotated mainly by the action of the popliteus and semitendinosus. These small movements play an important role in the overall function of the knee joint but tend not to be movements that we intentionally focus on during a yoga practice.

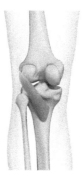

Popliteus

There are no muscles that perform medial and lateral (valgus and varus) movements of the knee. These movements originate from the hip joint or the ankle joint. The tensor fasciae latae and iliotibial band (which we will explore in the next chapter) resist lateral (varus) movement of the knee joint while the sartorius, gracilis and semitendinosus muscles resist medial (valgus) movement.

DEMYSTIFYING HYPEREXTENSION OR 'LOCKING' OF THE KNEE JOINT

The terms hyperextension and locking of the knee joint each have different meanings depending on the context. In the medical world, knee hyperextension (or genu recurvatum) is a deformity in the knee joint where excessive extension occurs and the knee bends backwards. In terms of anatomical language hyperextension of the knee is simply extending the knee beyond 180°. In the fitness world the term 'locking' the knee is often used interchangeably with hyperextension. This phrase actually refers to the 'screw-home' mechanism involving lateral rotation that occurs at full extension of the knee to create stability.

There is very limited literature regarding hyperextension of the knee joint. Gray *et al.* (2005) stated that overextension of the knee joint is prevented by the tension of the anterior cruciate, oblique popliteal and collateral ligaments, while Morgan *et al.* (2010) shared that the oblique popliteal ligament specifically limits hyperextension of the knee. We will discuss some of these ligaments in the next section. Loudon, Goist and Loudon (1998) stated that with knee hyperextension the femur tilts forward relative to the tibia creating anterior compression between the femur and tibia. In this position, the posterior structures are placed in tension, which helps to stabilize the knee joint, and no quadriceps muscle activity is necessary. This can be seen in individuals following a cerebral vascular accident who lose motor control of the quadriceps and are still able to stand. Therefore it can be concluded that in a standing position when the knee is hyperextended we bear weight using the strength of these knee ligaments and not the knee musculature.

We will look at some of the potential advantages and disadvantages associated with hyperextending the knee joint later in the chapter.

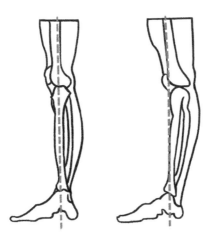

Knee extension versus hyperextension

The main knee ligaments

There are many ligaments in the knee joint, but we are going to focus on the two main pairs: the collateral ligaments and the cruciate ligaments.

The medial collateral ligament (MCL) provides stability to the medial aspect of the knee, preventing excessive valgus stress during external rotation of the knee, becoming tight during extension and external rotation, and becoming loose during flexion and internal rotation. The lateral collateral ligament (LCL) runs from the femur to the fibula to stabilize the lateral aspect of the knee, preventing excessive varus stress and external rotation at all positions of knee flexion (Gollehon, Torzilli and Warren 1987). By contraction of the biceps femoris tendon, the LCL is actively tightened (Mueller 1982).

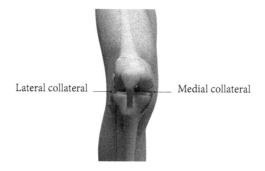

Lateral collateral ———   ——— Medial collateral

Collateral ligaments

The name cruciate originates from the Latin word for 'cross' since the ligaments cross each other when viewed from the side. The anterior cruciate ligament (ACL) attaches to the anterior surface of the tibia, prevents anterior dislocation of the tibia in relation to the femur and also limits knee rotation. The ACL is considered the main stabilizer of the knee, contributing to about 85% of the knee stabilization and enabling smooth and stable flexion and rotation of the knee (Ellison and Berg 1985). The posterior cruciate ligament (PCL) attaches to the posterior surface of the tibia and prevents posterior dislocation of the tibia in relation to the femur. Both the ACL and PCL assist the collateral ligaments in resisting varus and valgus stress.

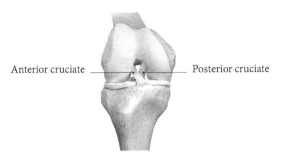

Anterior cruciate — — Posterior cruciate

Cruciate ligaments

THE NOCEBO EFFECT AND
FEAR-BASED LANGUAGE

I imagine that most of us are familiar with the placebo effect. It is a phenomenon that has been proven countless times through scientific research that tells us that if we have a positive expectation of an event, we are more likely to experience a positive outcome. If you have high blood pressure and are given a tablet every day that you believe to be the most effective medication for reducing blood pressure the likelihood is that your blood pressure will lower, even if the tablet is in fact an M&M.

Did you know that the opposite is also true? It's called the nocebo effect and this phenomenon tells us that a negative expectation of an otherwise harmless event can lead to a negative outcome (Planès, Villier and Mallaret 2016). So, if you were given a tablet for high blood pressure but told that it was just an M&M, your blood pressure would not lower significantly even if the tablet was a very effective medication for lowering blood pressure.

Your brain and nervous system are hardwired at a primal level to be on the lookout all the time for anything that is threatening. That threat may come in the form of an injury, in the words someone says to you or even what you read online about the human body.

Nocebic[1] language is everywhere, particularly in the medical world. Think about the term 'chronic pain'. The term chronic

---

1   I have used some artist license with the word nocebic.

essentially means permanent even though no experience is ever permanent. Even someone who experiences persistent pain doesn't experience the pain at every moment. Another term is 'treatment-resistant depression' referring to depression that has not responded to three treatments. How would you feel if you had depression and were then told that you were treatment resistant?

This language can also appear frequently in a yoga class setting: 'Keep your knee above your ankle in Warrior Pose to *protect* your knee', 'Keep your knee in line with your ankle to *protect* your knee', 'Place your foot above or below your knee in Tree Pose but not against it', 'Micro-bend your standing leg to *protect* your knee' and 'Flex your foot in Pigeon Pose to *protect* your knee' to name just a few.

These statements are not only fear based but are also generally false and can't be backed up with sound anatomical logic. I believe that the origin of this stems from a general lack of anatomical, physiological and biomechanical knowledge. We are often taught that our knees are simply hinge joints that move in one plane. No wonder so many of us don't want our students to put lateral force on the knee joint. Our knee joints are in fact much more complex than this as we have started to discuss. Our bodies are also *anti-fragile* which means that our tissues strengthen when stressed appropriately. But if you believe that your knees are fragile, and this message gets reinforced time and time again, then you are more likely to experience pain and dysfunction in your knees.

Let's change the narrative that has been created around the knee joint. Look after your knees, move them well and move them often. Listen to your body and respond if there is feedback. But please don't imagine that your knees are fragile.

The phrase 'Keep your knee above your ankle to protect your knee' could be replaced with: 'In the pose we generally keep the knee above the ankle.'

The menisci

Each knee has two fibrocartilaginous discs called menisci that are positioned medially and laterally. The primary function of the meniscus is to transmit load across the knee joint by increasing congruency and therefore decrease the resultant stress placed on the hyaline cartilage. The menisci also play a secondary role in shock absorption, stability, lubrication, nutrition and proprioception to the knee joint (Englund, Guermazi and Lohmander 2009).

The lateral meniscus is much more mobile than the medial one, which means that it can better compensate for rotational forces. The medial meniscus receives a greater blood supply than the lateral meniscus: only 10–30% of the medial meniscus border and 10–25% of the lateral meniscus border receives direct blood supply (Arnoczky and Warren 1982) while the remaining portion of each meniscus (65–75%) receives nourishment only from the synovial fluid via diffusion (Mow, Fithian and Kelly 1989). Both menisci have connections with the ACL and PCL.

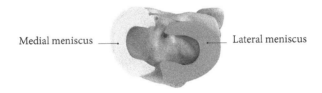

Medial meniscus ——— Lateral meniscus

Superior view of right menisci

The bursae

The knee has many bursae, which are fluid-filled cavities located at tissue sites that facilitate movement of the tendons and skin over the joint. They are filled with synovial fluid and help in reducing friction between adjacent moving structures. They are distributed around high-motion areas to ensure smooth, friction-free movement.

The Q-angle

The orientation of the quadriceps muscle force is expressed in terms of the Q-angle and was first described by Brattström (1964). The Q-angle approximates the resultant force orientation of the four muscles of the quadriceps group acting on the patella. The Q-angle is defined as the angle between a line connecting the center of the patella and the patellar tendon attachment site on the tibial tubercle, and a second line connecting the center of the patella and the anterior superior iliac spine on the pelvis when the knee is fully extended.

There are no universally accepted normal or abnormal values of the Q-angle, which may be due in part to the absence of a standardized measurement position. A study by Emami *et al.* (2007) established 13.5° ± 4.5° as the mean Q-angle for healthy subjects between the ages of 18 and 35 years, regardless of gender. They found that the mean Q-angle for women is 4.6° higher than that for men.

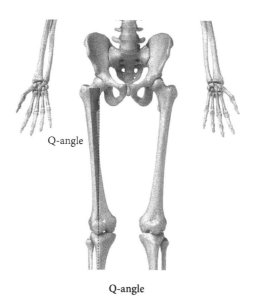

Q-angle

Genu valgum and genu varum

Tetsworth and Paley (1994) stated that alignment in the lower limb is determined by the line extending from the center of the hip joint to the center of the ankle joint. This can be referred to as the mechanical axis or weight-bearing line of the limb and malalignment can be thought of as the center of the knee joint not lying close to this line. This is best judged by radiography.

In genu varum (bow-leg), this line passes medial to the knee and increases the force across the medial compartment. In genu valgum (knock-knee), the load-bearing axis passes lateral to the knee and increases the force across the lateral compartment (Levangie and Norkin 2005).

Both genu valgum and genu varum are commonly reported knee joint deformities and are more frequent in women (Kendall *et al.* 2005).

Genu varum develops as a normal variation in many toddlers, straightening at around two years of age and reversing into genu valgum at approximately three years of age. This is then typically followed by gradual reduction of genu valgum to the normal adult level of 5° to 7° by six to seven years of age (Lee, Perez-Rossello and Weissman 2009). Genu valgus may also be seen in early adolescence, when it is thought to be a result of rapid growth.

The underlying causes of genu varum and genu valgum are often complicated and rarely clearly understood. Both muscular imbalances and specific bony architectures can play a significant role. Carreiro (2009) stated that chronic contraction of the hip adductor muscles, weakness of the external hip rotator muscles, flatfoot, everted calcaneus, an internally rotated femur, internally rotated tibia and/or an anteriorly tipped pelvis can lead to genu valgum in children. It is fair to say that the opposite may then be true for genu varum.

Relating this to yoga, it is important to note that the common principle of keeping the knee in line with the center of the ankle in such poses as Chair Pose (Utkatasana) becomes arbitrary. This principle will work well for some students who lie in the middle of the knee alignment spectrum but will not work so well for all the students who lie off-center on the spectrum. I might phrase this by saying to my students, 'In this pose we generally keep the knees tracking in line with the ankles, but this won't work for everyone's anatomy. Let's focus more on how our knees feel in this pose, making adaptations when we need to.'

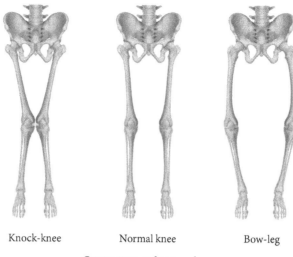

Knock-knee   Normal knee   Bow-leg

Genu varum and genu valgum

Common knee injuries and conditions

In this section we will explore some of the most common knee injuries and conditions that affect our population.

Osteoarthritis (OA)

Sometimes called degenerative joint disease or 'wear and tear' arthritis, OA is one of the most common joint disorders worldwide (Cross *et al.* 2014) and is characterized by pain, swelling and stiffness. The reported prevalence and incidence rates of OA vary widely but knee OA has been noted to be the most common type, affecting 6% of all adults (Andrianakos *et al.* 2006). The absence of lymphatics, nerve endings and blood vessels in the hyaline cartilage does not allow its regeneration (Umlauf *et al.* 2010).

The risk factors of OA can be divided into person-level factors, including age, gender, obesity, genetics and diet, and joint-level factors, including injury and abnormal loading of the joints (Johnson and Hunter 2014). The disease is more common in women than men and the incidence increases with age, occurring after 40–50 years of age (Palazzo *et al.* 2016).

The rupture of the ACL leads to early-onset knee OA in 13% of cases after 10–15 years. When such rupture is associated with damaged cartilage, bone, collateral ligaments and/or menisci, the prevalence of knee OA is higher, between 21% and 40% (Øiestad *et al.* 2009; Slauterbeck *et al.* 2009). Knee OA was more frequently observed in people with occupations that required squatting and kneeling (Croft *et al.* 1992). Highly repetitive, intense and high-impact physical activity seems to confer increased risk of developing radiographic knee OA as compared with controls, but it is unclear whether this association is only due to sports participation or results from injury (Johnson and Hunter 2014). Hunter *et al.* (2007) and Palazzo *et al.* (2016) suggested that malalignment is not a risk factor for OA, but rather is a marker of disease severity and/or its progression.

There is a strong dissociation between radiographic findings and clinical symptoms: in 1988 Anderson and Felson found that only 40% of patients with moderate radiographic knee OA and 60% of those with severe knee OA have symptoms, while in 2000 Hannan, Felson and Pincus found that only about 15% of patients with radiologically demonstrated knee OA complain of knee pain.

Prevention here is key: if the influences that can potentially damage the knee are eliminated early enough then the development of OA can be prevented, or at least the progression of any changes that are already present can be slowed.

Moseley *et al.* (2002) reported that 180 people with painful knee OA randomized to either arthroscopic lavage (a visually guided 'wash out' of the knee joint), arthroscopic debridement (basically filing down rough knee cartilage) or placebo surgery (skin incisions) had the same improvement at two-year follow-up. This strongly suggests that the benefit reported for people undergoing arthroscopic surgery for painful degenerative knees may be entirely attributable to the placebo effect.

Chondromalacia patella

Sometimes referred to as 'runner's knee', chondromalacia patella is an inflammation or persistent irritation of the posterior surface of the patella. The distinguishing characteristic is softening of the cartilage, and patients sometimes also report a grinding sensation. The patella cartilage acts as a natural shock absorber, and once erosion occurs and the surface is no longer smooth, movement can become painful. Chondromalacia patella is far more common than is generally believed, because usually it does not cause symptoms (Outerbridge and Outerbridge 2001).

A study of the literature on chondromalacia patella showed that its etiology is poorly understood. It may occur due to an acute injury, after knee surgery or after overuse from participating in high-activity sports. Insall, Falvo and Wise (1976) suggested that lateral positioning of the patella in the patella-femoral joint is a frequent cause of chondromalacia, with an abnormal Q-angle often being the cause.

Patellofemoral pain syndrome (PFPS)

PFPS is defined as diffuse pain around or behind the patella, which is aggravated by activities that load the patellofemoral joint, such as squatting, running, jumping and ascending and descending stairs. The term is used rather broadly but differs from chondromalacia in that there is no cartilage damage. Symptoms include crepitus (joint noises), tenderness on palpation of the patella edges and pain upon straightening the knee following sitting.

It is the most common cause of knee pain in female athletes and is a result of imbalances in the forces controlling patellar tracking during knee flexion and extension (Rixe *et al.* 2013). Females are twice as likely to develop PFPS than males (Taunton *et al.* 2002).

Genu valgum, knee hyperextension, Q-angle and excessive hindfoot pronation are some of the alignment factors that have been associated with PFPS (Thomee, Augustsson and Karlsson 1999). A number of muscular imbalances are also thought to contribute to PFPS development including decreased knee extensor strength, imbalance between the vastus medialis and vastus lateralis components of the quadriceps, and hip muscle weakness (Pattyn *et al.* 2001).

Collateral ligament injuries

The MCL is the most commonly injured ligament in the knee, affecting males twice as frequently as females. The majority of MCL tears are isolated and these injuries occur predominantly in young individuals participating in sports activities such as skiing, ice hockey and soccer.

The mechanism of injury involves valgus knee loading and/or external rotation (Wijdicks *et al.* 2010).

The MCL has the greatest healing potential of any ligament in the knee (Fanelli and Harris 2006) and it is generally accepted that most partial and isolated MCL injuries can be treated non-operatively with early functional rehabilitation (Ballmer and Jakob 1988). In sports injuries the MCL is involved seven times more often (17.5%) than the LCL (2.5%) (Majewski, Susanne and Klaus 2006).

Cruciate ligament injuries

ACL injuries are common, and the incidence continues to increase in both the general population and individuals who play sports. Football players sustain the greatest number of ACL injuries (53% of the total) with skiers and gymnasts also at high risk. ACL injury rates tend to be higher for women than for men (Siegel, Vandenakker-Albanese and Siegel 2012). Anatomic features, such as a decrease in femoral notch width, a decrease in the depth of concavity of the medial tibial plateau and an increase in the posterior-inferior-directed (backward and downward) slope of the tibial plateau, may act in combination to increase the risk of suffering an ACL injury (Smith *et al.* 2012).

A 2012 study by Nordenvall *et al.* suggested that 36% of patients with an ACL injury undergo surgery. When the ACL is torn the blood supply is usually permanently disrupted and reconstruction is the preferred surgical choice (Flandry and Hommel 2011).

PCL injuries are much less common than ACL injuries. A ten-year study by Majewski *et al.* (2006) found that incidence rates for ACL injuries were over 30 times greater than PCL injuries. Unlike the ACL, blood supply is not permanently lost with a tear of the PCL and primary repair of these injuries is possible (Flandry and Hommel 2011). Repair keeps the native ligament, while reconstruction completely replaces the native ligament.

Meniscal tears

Coupled compressive and rotational knee joint forces can produce injuries to a healthy meniscus. These forces tend to pinch the menisci as they attempt to rapidly conform to the three-dimensional joint stresses. These coupled forces commonly occur during athletic movements that require sudden directional changes (Wheatley, Krome and Martin 1996). Stocker *et al.* (1997) reported that meniscal injuries accounted for 12% of all football knee injuries. However, older patients may present without a specific mechanism of injury as their meniscal injuries are often due to degenerative processes. We can generally categorize the mechanism of injury of meniscal tears as occurring during a sporting activity (e.g., soccer, rugby or football), a non-sporting activity (e.g., squatting) or non-activity. Drosos and Pozo (2004) found that only one-third of patients incurred their meniscal injury in a sports-related activity, while over one-third of the injuries occurred due to non-sporting activities and nearly one-third of patients could not identify any specific event or incident which resulted in an injury.

As mentioned earlier, the lateral meniscus is much more mobile than the medial one, which means that it can better compensate for rotational forces, but the medial meniscus receives a greater blood supply than the lateral meniscus. This is reflected by the higher rate of medial meniscus tears but longer rehabilitation timeline for lateral meniscus tears (Hirschmann and Müller 2015). Meniscus injuries are observed in approximately 65–75% of ACL-injured knees (Palazzo *et al.* 2016) with lateral meniscus tears being more common.

Felson *et al.* (2013) suggested that valgus malalignment is a potent cause of lateral meniscal damage while Englund *et al.* (2011) suggested that varus malalignment increases the risk of medial meniscal tears.

Bursitis

Bursitis is inflammation of the bursae with precipitating factors including infections, rheumatoid arthritis, trauma or minor injuries. Bursitis tends not to have a direct structural effect on joint stability. Conservative measures, such as rest and icing, often help.

The pes bursa is a synovial-lined sac that lies deep to the pes anserinus (conjoined tendon of the sartorius, gracilis and semitendinosus) and superficial to the tibial attachment of the MCL. Bursitis at this site typically presents as medial knee pain, which usually increases with exercise and is felt about two to three inches below the medial knee. It can be the result of overuse, sudden exertion, tight hamstrings, obesity or other factors that put stress on the knee (Grover and Rakhra 2010).

Other common sites of bursitis in the knee include the deep infrapatellar bursa due to its vital role in preventing friction between the patellar tendon and the tibia, and the gastrocnemius-semimembranosus bursa (located between the medial femoral condyle, semimembranosus tendon and the medial head of the gastrocnemius). The latter is often called a Baker's or popliteal cyst.

JOINT NOISES

Joint noises are very common and are referred to as crepitus in the medical world. The exact cause of the sounds that our joints make is not always completely understood. There is agreement in the literature regarding the formation of a bubble as part of the mechanism of some joint crepitus; however, the process by which the bubble is formed and the source of the cracking sound are not clear. There is also suggestion that the noise might be coming from different soft tissue structures coming into contact with each other.

There is no research that I am aware of that has demonstrated a definitive link between joint noise and pathology. McCoy *et al.* (1987) demonstrated that 99% of a cohort of subjects with no knee pain had patellofemoral crepitus. Robertson (2010) suggested that crepitus is often present in the complete absence of any joint pathology.

A study by Robertson, Hurley and Jones (2017) suggested that patients often hold negative beliefs about their crepitus and in turn this may negatively affect their behavior. Amongst participants there was a common belief that crepitus denoted degeneration and enhanced feelings of premature aging. Participants reported that the noise made them feel old, and at times this led them to be less active.

A helpful guide is that if you are not experiencing pain or any other symptoms along with the sounds then this is most likely a sign of a normal, healthy joint. If pain or other symptoms accompany the sounds, then advice from a medical professional should be sought.

Key yoga asanas and how to adapt them

We will now explore some asanas that may present a challenge to students who are affected by the common injuries or conditions that we have discussed above and look at some of the ways that these can be adapted in order to make them more accessible.

Limiting knee rotation

Hero Pose (Virasana) might not be a great option for a student who has a knee injury or condition. Some options here include raising the seat with a bolster or foam block, taking Saddle Pose with the knees wide and big toes touching to limit rotational movement in the knee or simply finding any other seated position that feels more accessible.

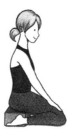

Hero Pose

Pigeon Pose (Eka Pada Rajakapotasana) is often classified as a 'hip opener'. We will discuss this phrase in the next chapter. To avoid the pose becoming a 'knee opener' we need to look at how the action of the ankle joint can impact the knee joint in this position. When the front foot and ankle are relaxed and weight-bearing in this asana, both the ankle joint and knee joint can experience significant lateral force. To avoid this, it is a good idea to activate the front foot and ankle by spreading across the toes and resisting the natural inversion position of the ankle by pressing the part of the foot that is in contact with the mat down into the mat. I think of these actions as creating an 'active foot' as opposed to a passive one. By engaging the musculature of the foot and lower leg we can limit the rotational movement of the knee joint and focus the movement on the hip joint instead, which is the real focus of the pose. The position of the front ankle in terms of dorsiflexion or plantar flexion is an individual choice and will depend on what feels best for the student. Supine Pigeon Pose is a great alternative here with very similar benefits to be had but much less pressure placed on the front knee.

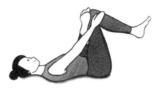

Supine Pigeon Pose

If your knees are not feeling happy in Warrior 2 (Virabhadrasana II) start by finding a narrower stance. Try stepping your feet apart in the frontal plane rather than lining your heels up along the length of your mat. A great alternative position is High Lunge where your back heel is lifted and pointing directly behind you. This position makes it easier to turn the front of your pelvis forward and avoids rotation in your back knee. A chair can also be placed under the front thigh to provide support or the asana can be practiced while sitting at the edge of a chair.

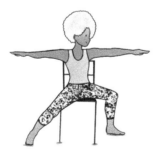

Warrior 2

Lotus Pose (Padmasana) is inaccessible to most yoga practitioners mainly due to the bony architecture of their hip joints. We will explore the fact that every body is unique in more detail in the next chapter. Lotus Pose requires a significant range of movement in external rotation, and hips that lack this range can easily refer strong rotational tension to the knee joint. If in doubt, simply avoid this pose. Find an alternative sitting position, or if you are wanting to specifically access hip mobility try Supine Pigeon Pose.

Limiting knee hyperextension

For Extended Triangle Pose (Trikonasana) a narrow stance is often a great option. Placing the front hand on a chair helps to reduce some of the load placed on the knee joints. Keeping the core engaged can have a positive impact on the leg musculature and make avoiding hyperextension of the knees more accessible. In the next section we will discuss how to 'co-contract' the knee musculature in this pose.

Some helpful suggestions for Tree Pose (Vriksasana) include practicing this asana with the lifted foot against the ankle and the tips of the toes connected to the ground instead of taking the foot higher up the standing leg. Placing hands on the hips keeps the center of gravity lower and this will be a big help too. A wall, pillar or chair could also be used for support here.

Kneeling positions

In a Low Lunge position placing a blanket under the length of the back shinbone not only provides cushioning but also allows the student to spread the weight-bearing load over a larger surface.

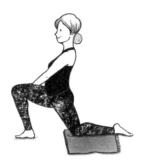

Low Lunge

In Camel Pose (Ustrasana) folding the yoga mat over and/or kneeling on a blanket can add necessary cushioning. Pressing the length of the shinbones into the mat can again help to spread the weight-bearing load while squeezing a block between the thighs can help to create more lift in the pose.

Deep knee flexion

In Child's Pose (Balasana) good options include placing a small rolled-up towel behind the knees to provide some cushioning or placing a bolster between the thighs to keep the pelvis raised slightly. Supine Child's Pose is an alternative option here. If the purpose of this pose is to allow for a moment of rest and integration then any position that feels restful is a great option.

In Garland Pose (Malasana) placing blocks under the heels can help a lot of students to create more lift and action. A good support is to sit on a stack of wide yoga blocks to raise the seat. Goddess Pose (Utkata Konasana) can be a more accessible alternative to this pose.

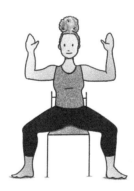

Goddess Pose

Improving the overall health of the knee joint

This section addresses some effective ways in which we can all improve and maintain the health and functioning of our knees. It is intended to be a general guide for yoga practitioners and teachers and is not a replacement for the personal advice of a health professional.

The position of the knee between the two longest lever arms of the body, the femur and tibia, means that the foot and ankle and the hip joint have a huge impact on the knee joint. Therefore, all of the foot and ankle exercises that we discussed in the previous chapter and all of the hip exercises that we will discuss in the next chapter will play a big role when looking at improving the health of the knee joint.

Knee hyperextension

In an ideal scenario hyperextension of the knee should be a choice that we are making and not just the default knee position that we adopt. Become more aware of how you stand during your day and start to notice when you might be hyperextending your knee.

Earlier in the chapter we concluded that in a standing position when the knee is hyperextended, we bear weight using the strength of the knee ligaments and not the knee musculature. It is best to avoid knee hyperextension during your asana practice if you are rehabilitating from a knee injury or if it feels painful to do so. Taking the knee joint into its end range of extension can make it more challenging to effectively engage the muscles around the joint, therefore limiting our ability to increase the strength of these muscles.

It might well be appropriate to choose to hyperextend the knee joint during your asana practice if you intend to stress the ligaments of the knee in order to strengthen them. Davis's law states that by stressing connective tissue we strengthen it, while lack of use can lead to weakness and atrophy. The stress that is applied needs to be progressive. It is a good idea to explore hyperextension in a seated asana like Staff Pose (Dandasana) where your legs are stretched out in front of you. Engage your quadriceps to lift the patella and notice if your heels begin to lift off the mat. Take note of how this feels.

Co-contraction of the knee musculature

We will now discuss how we can gain the awareness and strength to resist hyperextension if that feels like the right choice for us.

1.   Sit on your mat with your legs stretched out in front of you.

2. You can always raise your seat with a cushion if it is challenging to keep your spine long.

3. Bring your awareness to your quadriceps at the front of your thighs.

4. Engage these by pulling your kneecaps up towards your torso.

5. You will notice that your heels may start to lift off the mat.

6. This action can be subtle or very obvious.

7. Now keep the engagement of your quadriceps as you press your heels back towards the mat.

8. This action simultaneously engages both the hamstrings and the quadriceps, 'hugging' the knee joint and preventing hyperextension.

9. We can call this 'co-contraction'.

Once you have explored co-contraction in a seated position you can progress to trying it in a standing posture such as Extended Triangle Pose (Trikonasana).

1. Engage your quadriceps.

2. Notice the backs of your knees move back slightly as you move into knee hyperextension.

3. Now keep this engagement at the front of your thighs but energetically draw your feet towards each other (they won't actually move).

4. Your entire thigh will firm.

5. Repeat this on the other side.

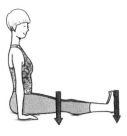

Co-contraction of the knee musculature

Chapter 3

THE HIP

The anatomy of the hip joint

The hip joint is a true ball-and-socket joint, enabling a wide range of motion in each plane while also exhibiting remarkable stability. The hip joints are the structural links between the lower limbs and the axial skeleton and therefore not only transmit forces from the ground up but also carry forces from the trunk, head and neck, and upper limbs.

The bony architecture of the hip joint

The bony components of the hip joint are the head of the femur and the acetabulum of the hip bone.

The femur is the longest and strongest bone in the human body. The proximal end of the femur consists of the head, neck and shaft. The greater trochanter and lesser trochanter are bony landmarks on the femur that serve as attachment points to many of the key muscles of the hip.

In the immature skeleton each hip bone is made up of three separate bones: the ilium, the ischium and the pubis. Fusion of these three bones starts to occur around the age of 14–16 years and is usually complete by the age of 23 (Moore 1992). The cup-shaped acetabulum, or hip socket, is formed at the area where these three bones meet.

The two hip bones join with the sacrum and the coccyx to form the bowl-shaped pelvis (Latin for basin). Some important bony landmarks on the pelvis include the ischial tuberosities ('sitting bones' or 'sitz bones'), the pubic symphysis formed by the union of the two pubic bones and the anterior superior iliac spine (ASIS). The pelvis is explored in much more detail in the next chapter.

Hyaline cartilage covers the head of the femur and creates a C-shaped ring around the acetabulum of the hip bone. It serves as a load-bearing elastic material that is responsible for the frictionless movement of the articulating surfaces and is therefore crucial for efficient functioning of the joint.

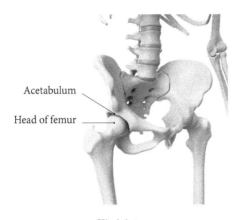

Acetabulum

Head of femur

Hip joint

The labrum and capsule

The labrum of the hip joint is a fibrocartilaginous rim attached to the margin of the acetabulum. The exact function of the labrum is not fully understood but it may act to protect the edge of the acetabulum and fill up the irregularities of its surface. The labrum may also be involved in load distribution and lubrication within the joint (Ferguson *et al.* 2003). It is much thicker above and behind than below and in front. The majority of the labrum is thought to be avascular. Studies have shown blood vessels entering primarily the peripheral part of the labrum, with penetration only into the outer one-third of the substance of the labrum (Lewis and Sahrmann 2006).

The articular capsule is a strong and dense structure that attaches to the margin of the acetabulum and wraps around the neck of the femur. While the ball-and-socket configuration naturally gives the hip joint great stability the capsule undoubtedly contributes significantly to this. Proprioceptive feedback (information about limb position and movement) is in part provided from receptors in the hip capsule (Torry *et al.* 2006).

The main ligaments of the hip joint

The transverse ligament is in reality a portion of the labrum, consisting of strong, flattened fibers, which cross the acetabular notch and convert it into a foramen through which vessels enter the joint.

The iliofemoral ligament is a band of great strength that lies in front of the joint running from the ASIS to the base of the neck of the femur. It is the strongest of all the ligaments in the body and is the main agent in keeping us upright without muscular fatigue by preventing the pelvis from posteriorly tilting. The iliofemoral ligament helps to limit hip extension, adduction (with flexion), abduction and external rotation.

The ischiofemoral ligament springs from the ischium below and behind the acetabulum, and blends with the joint capsule around the base of the neck of the femur. This ligament limits internal rotation of the hip joint.

The pubofemoral ligament, located on the inferior surface of the hip joint, extends from the pubic portion of the acetabular rim and passes below the neck of the femur. This ligament limits hip abduction.

The ligamentum teres runs from the central area of the femur head to the inferior margin of the acetabulum. Although traditional orthopedic teaching has been to regard the ligamentum teres as a redundant or vestigial structure in the adult hip, O'Donnell, Devitt and Arora (2018) stated that it acts as a secondary stabilizer of the hip, supplementing the role of the capsular ligaments, and works in a sling-like manner to prevent dislocation of the femoral head at the extremes of motion.

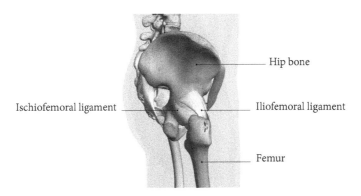

Ischiofemoral ligament

Hip bone

Iliofemoral ligament

Femur

Ligaments of the hip joint and pelvis

INTELLIGENT MOVEMENT PRINCIPLE – EVERY BODY IS UNIQUE

Have you ever wondered why certain yoga asanas can feel so ease-ful in your body while other asanas can feel like such a challenge? Or why one person can sit cross-legged for hours having never practiced yoga before and you still need to sit on four cushions after having practiced yoga for years? The short answer to this is that every body is entirely unique, with a unique range of movement in each joint, and therefore we will each express a certain yoga pose in a completely unique way. Let's explore this further using our hip joints as an example.

Femoral neck-shaft angles show considerable variation within human populations. There are no universally accepted normal or abnormal angles. Anderson and Trinkaus (1998) stated that mean values range from 122° to 136°, and normal individuals are found from around 110° to almost 150°. Peelle *et al.* (2005) stated that coxa vara is the condition when the neck-shaft angle is less than 126° and coxa valga is the condition when the angle is greater than 139°. Relating this natural variation to yoga, the femoral neck-shaft angle will impact the degree to which one can move one's leg directly out to the side (abduction) in a pose like Wide Leg Forward Fold (Prasarita Padottanasana).

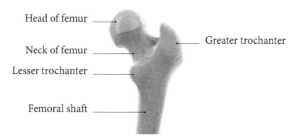

Head of femur

Greater trochanter

Neck of femur

Lesser trochanter

Femoral shaft

Posterior view of the right femur

The femoral neck in the average person is also rotated slightly anterior and this is referred to as femoral anteversion (AV). Bråten, Terjesen and Rossvoll (1992) found significant variation amongst the group in their study and state that the mean AV angle was 18° in the women and 14° in the men. The mean left/right difference in AV was 3.8°. The AV angle will inevitably impact the range of movement of the hip joint in flexion, extension and rotation.

The size, shape and orientation of the lesser and greater trochanter can also play a big role in impacting the range of movement.

The bony structure of the acetabulum varies immensely from person to person. While one yoga student may have a shallow acetabulum, another student may have a much deeper socket. This variation can impact the range of movement of the hip joint in all directions. The actual position of the acetabulum on the hip bone also varies immensely. Some people have an acetabulum that is positioned slightly further forward on the hip bone or further back, angled upward or downward. There are an infinite number of possibilities here.

Our bodies are not naturally symmetrical. No one has a right hip joint that is architecturally identical to the left hip joint. This means that our right hip joint will always have a different range of movement compared to the left. While practicing Extended Triangle Pose (Trikonasana) easily on the right we might find that there is a sense of compression in the left hip that requires us to step our feet closer together to overcome.

Yoga is a wonderful practice for developing a deep sense of awareness of our bodies and is a powerful way to move towards accepting our limitations and celebrating our uniqueness.

The hip joint movements and musculature

There are 22 muscles that act on the hip joint and allow it to move in each of the three planes.

The musculature of the hip and thigh is wrapped in a continuous fibrous layer called the fascia lata. Its inelasticity functions to limit bulging of the thigh muscles, thus improving the efficiency of their contractions (Moore 1992). We will explore these muscles depending on the main movements of the hip joint that they help perform. It is important to note that they can contribute to movement in several different planes depending on the position of the hip, which is caused by a change in the relationship between the line of action of a muscle and the axis of rotation of the hip.

The most superficial muscle that is involved in external rotation of the hip is gluteus maximus. It is the largest muscle in the body and its size is one of the most characteristic features of human anatomy given that it allows us to be bipedal (stand and walk on two limbs). Gluteus maximus is also the most powerful extensor of the hip joint along with the hamstrings group.

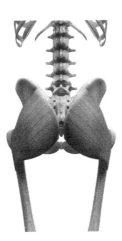

Gluteus maximus

There are six deeper muscles that also play a key role in external rotation: piriformis, quadratus femoris, gemellus inferior and superior, and obturator internus and externus. The six deep external rotators are all short muscles that insert on the greater trochanter of the femur. Piriformis runs laterally from the pelvic surface of the sacrum. When the hip is extended it externally rotates the joint, but when the hip is flexed it internally rotates the joint. Obturator internus and piriformis can also be thought of as being part of the pelvic floor, which we will explore in more detail in the next chapter.

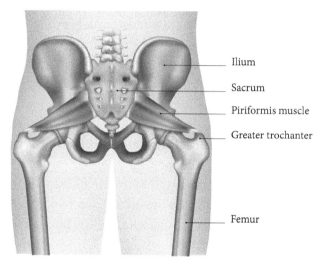

Ilium

Sacrum

Piriformis muscle

Greater trochanter

Femur

Piriformis

The main muscles involved in internal hip rotation are gluteus medius, gluteus minimus and tensor fascia lata (TFL). The TFL runs from the ASIS and inserts into the iliotibial band (ITB). Deep to this muscle lies gluteus medius, which runs from the iliac crest of the hip bone to the greater trochanter of the femur. Gluteus minimus is deep again to gluteus medius, arising from the gluteal surface of the ilium and inserting on the greater trochanter. Gluteus medius, gluteus minimus and TFL are also the main muscles involved in abduction of the hip when the hip is extended.

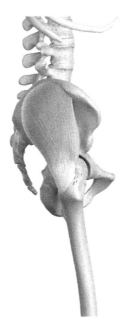

Gluteus medius

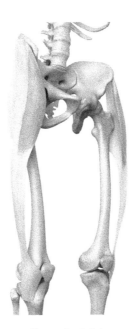

Tensor fascia lata

The hip adductors (pectineus, adductor brevis, adductor longus, adductor magnus and gracilis) originate in the region of the pubic bone and insert on the distal femur.

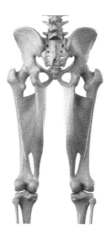

Adductor magnus

The main flexors of the hip joint are iliopsoas, rectus femoris and sartorius. Iliopsoas comprises of iliacus, psoas minor and psoas major. Psoas major arises from the vertebral bodies of T12–L5 and is joined by the iliacus to insert into the lesser trochanter of the femur. Psoas major is important for sitting in an erect position and stability of the spine in the frontal plane, and iliacus is important for stabilizing the pelvis (Andersson *et al.* 1995). Psoas minor is absent in a large percentage of the population (Farias *et al.* 2012).

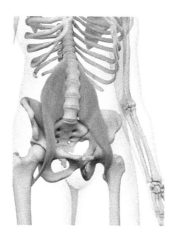

Psoas major

MUSCLE MISCONCEPTIONS

There are many assumptions made about changes in muscle length from calf muscles lengthening from practicing Downward Facing Dog (Adho Mukha Svanasana) to hamstrings and hip flexors shortening with prolonged sitting. While traditionally literature has attributed increases in muscle extensibility observed after stretching to a mechanical increase in muscle length, a review by Weppler and Magnusson (2010) reported that a growing body of research refutes these mechanical theories, suggesting instead that the increases in muscle extensibility observed are predominantly due to modification in subjects' sensation (often referred to as 'stretch tolerance'). Findings from this review also suggest that muscles labeled as 'shortened' are lacking in extensibility rather than being short in terms of physical structure. A study by Krabak *et al.* (2001) examined the passive range of movement in patients before, during and after anesthesia and found that this increased significantly during anesthesia. This not only implicates nervous system contributions to muscle extensibility but also refutes the concept of 'shortened' muscle tissue.

There also tend to be many assumptions made about muscle tightness. Tightness is a very vague term that means different things to different people. When someone talks about muscle tightness, they could be referring to a lack of extensibility of a muscle and the associated decreased range of movement, a dull ache in the region, 'knots' felt in muscle or even a sense of energetic congestion. There are many potential causes of muscle tightness and for most of us the exact root often remains unclear. Overusing a muscle group, underusing a muscle group, trauma and/or injury and psychological stress can all play a role here. It is also important to recognize that the human body is a tensile structure and we rely on tension to resist the force of gravity and to perform everyday tasks. So, while the words tension and tightness often have a negative connotation, they can have very significant functions. If we begin to alter our internal dialogue around tightness and take a more holistic approach to unwanted tightness by stretching, strengthening and decreasing our stress levels we might well notice that our perceived levels of tightness decrease.

The main hip bursae

The iliopsoas bursa is positioned between the iliopsoas tendon and the bony surfaces of the pelvis and proximal femur. It has been shown to be the largest bursa in the human body (Tatu *et al.* 2001).

The trochanteric bursa is located beneath the gluteus maximus muscle and the iliotibial tract. The subgluteus medius bursa is deep in the distal gluteus medius tendon. The subgluteus minimus bursa lies beneath the gluteus minimus tendon.

WHAT EXACTLY DO WE MEAN BY 'HIP OPENING'?

The term 'hip opening' is used a lot in yoga but no one ever talks about what it is that we are attempting to open. What most people associate with this term is external rotation of the hip joint. Therefore the 'hip opener' category includes Warrior 1 (Virabhadrasana I), Cobbler's Pose (Baddha Konasana), Pigeon Pose (Eka Pada Rajakapotasana) and Easy Pose (Sukhasana), to name just a few. So many yoga asanas involve external hip rotation.

External rotation is an important movement of the hip and a lot of students have a limited range of movement here, but all of the other movements of the hip are just as important to focus on. In my experience most students tend to complain of 'tightness' in each direction of their hip movement but ways to explore our full range of active internal rotation of the hip joint, for example, are often missing from many asana sequences. So, let's try to focus equally on all hip movements, including adding in some targeted strengthening work, and we'll be on the way to healthier and happier hip joints.

Common hip injuries and conditions

In this section we will explore some of the most common hip injuries and conditions that affect our population.

Osteoarthritis (OA)

We have already discussed OA in the previous chapter related to the knee joint, but we will now discuss it in relation to the hip joint. Hip OA is a common cause of musculoskeletal pain in older adults that is characterized by destruction of articular cartilage and reactive bone changes and is associated clinically with regional pain, stiffness and dysfunction. It has been identified as one of the most common causes of debilitating pain in the general population (Ingvarsson 2000).

OA is generally considered a multifactorial disease that involves a combination of systemic risk factors (e.g., age, gender, hormone levels, genetics and nutrition), intrinsic joint risk factors (e.g., anatomical variants, muscle weakness, misalignment and joint laxity) and extrinsic risk factors (e.g., repetitive physical activities and obesity) (Dagenais, Garbedian and Wai 2009).

In a study by Croft *et al.* (1992) hip OA was more frequently observed in people with occupations associated with prolonged lifting and standing. Johnson and Hunter (2014) suggested that highly repetitive, intense and high-impact physical activity seems to be linked to an increased risk of developing radiographic hip OA as compared with controls, but whether this association is due to only sports participation or results from injury is unclear.

Developmental dysplasia of the hip (DDH)

The term DDH describes a spectrum of disorders that results in abnormal development of the hip joint. This spectrum can range from mild dysplasia of the acetabulum or femur to subluxation and high dislocation of the hip joint. If not treated successfully in childhood, these patients may go on to develop hip pathologies in adulthood. DDH commonly presents as a gradual onset of activity-related groin pain or lateral hip pain in young adults.

In patients with DDH, the labrum may undergo hypertrophy to increase the relative volume of acetabulum. Because of abnormal contact forces in patients with dysplasia, the labrum can also undergo degenerative changes and can tear (Parvizi *et al.* 2009).

DDH is the most common cause of secondary OA in young adults and this is thought to be a result of increased contact stresses (Kosuge *et al.* 2013).

Femoroacetabular impingement (FAI) syndrome

FAI syndrome is a relatively common non-arthritic cause of hip pain in young adults. Griffin *et al.* (2016) defined FAI syndrome as a motion-related clinical disorder of the hip with a triad of symptoms, clinical signs and imaging findings. It represents symptomatic premature contact between the femur and the acetabulum, and this phenomenon is associated with certain hip joint shapes.

The primary symptom of FAI syndrome is motion- or position-related pain in the hip or groin. Pain may also be felt in the back, buttock or thigh. Patients may also describe clicking, catching, locking, stiffness, restricted range of motion or giving way. There is often a limited range of hip motion, typically restricted internal rotation in flexion. The hip musculature is frequently weak in patients with FAI syndrome (Freke *et al.* 2016).

It is suggested that FAI syndrome accelerates the progression of hip OA (Ganz *et al.* 2003) although it is currently unknown whether treatment for FAI syndrome prevents hip OA.

Labral tears

Labral tears typically present with anterior hip or groin pain, and less commonly buttock pain; 71% of patients describe night pain (Hunt, Clohisy and Prather 2007).

A literature review by Groh and Herrera (2009) stated that the prevalence of labral tears in patients with hip or groin pain has been reported to be 22–55%; however, a study by Tresch *et al.* (2017) reported that 57% of 20–50-year-olds with no hip pain will have cartilage deducts and/or labral tears. Groh and Herrera (2009) reported that labral abnormalities have been found in patients without hip pain with the incidence increasing with age. This suggests that labral tears could be natural age-related changes.

A study by McCarthy *et al.* (2001) found that 86% of labral tears are located in the anterior quadrant and that 73% of patients with fraying or tearing of the acetabular labrum had cartilage damage.

The etiology of labral tears is believed to include trauma, FAI syndrome, capsular laxity/hip hypermobility, dysplasia and degeneration. In the athletic population up to 74.1% of labral tears are not associated with any known specific event or cause, and these are generally insidious in onset, with the underlying inciting event thought to be repetitive microtrauma (Groh and Herrera 2009).

IS MOVING BETWEEN INTERNAL AND EXTERNAL ROTATION ON A WEIGHT-BEARING HIP BAD FOR THE JOINT?

I have heard this topic mentioned a lot in the yoga sphere over the last few years and I suggest that the correlation between specific hip movements and hip pathology is anecdotal. To the best of my knowledge there are no studies that look at this specific topic. A study by Guanche and Sikka (2005) could not confirm an association between running and the development of labral tears or chondral lesions in the hip. As we have mentioned above, the etiology of most hip pathologies including labral tears is not clearly understood, and such changes may well be part of our natural aging process.

This means that it is really up to the individual to focus on how their hip joints feel in certain positions and during certain transitions. If moving from Warrior 3 (Virabhadrasana III) to Half Moon Pose (Ardha Chandrasana) with control feels okay then this transition will most likely be fine for the weight-bearing hip joint. If in doubt, come back to a neutral hip position before transitioning into the next asana.

Hamstring tendinopathies

Hamstring tendinopathies tend to be challenging injuries with persistent symptoms, slow healing and high reoccurrence rate. Strains usually occur in the biceps femoris and the most common location is near the muscle–tendon junction (Garrett 1996).

A literature review by Petersen and Hölmich (2005) stated that hamstring strains are amongst the most common injuries in sports that involve sprinting and jumping but are also common in dancing and waterskiing. They went on to state that the reoccurrence rate for hamstring injuries has been found to be between 12% and 31%.

The most common contributing factors have been found to be an imbalance of muscular strength with a low hamstring to quadriceps ratio, muscle fatigue, hamstring tightness, insufficient warm-up and previous injury (Petersen and Hölmich 2005). In a study of student ballet dancers by Askling *et al.* (2002) 88% of self-reported acute hamstring injuries occurred during slow activities in flexibility training.

Piriformis syndrome (PS)

PS is a poorly understood clinical syndrome involving buttock and leg pain. It is thought to be a nerve entrapment syndrome characterized by the entrapment of the sciatic nerve by the piriformis muscle. Hallin (1983) suggested that PS accounts for approximately 6–8% of sciatica.

A cadaver study by Beaton and Anson (1938) revealed that in 90% of cases the sciatic nerve emerges from below the piriformis. In 7% of cases the piriformis and the sciatic nerve are divided with one branch of the nerve passing through the split in the muscle and the other branch passing distal to the muscle. In 2% of cases only the sciatic nerve is divided.

Proposed causes of PS include overuse and hypertrophy of the piriformis, gluteal trauma, bursitis, and piriformis inflammation and spasticity (Jankovic, Peng and van Zundert 2013).

Bursitis

Trochanteric bursitis (TB) is characterized by chronic lateral hip pain exacerbated by active abduction, passive adduction and direct palpation. Although the incidence of TB is highest in middle-aged to elderly adults the etiology is multifactorial, and TB can affect patients of all ages (Lievense *et al.* 2005). The iliotibial band and fascia lata are often implicated as the source of TB.

Iliopsoas bursitis typically presents as anterior hip pain worsened by activity and/or a groin mass. The anterior hip pain may be referred to the abdomen, thigh or knee as a result of femoral nerve entrapment and may lead to a shortened stride on the affected side. To relieve pain, patients may passively hold their hip in flexion, adduction and external rotation, because this decreases tension of the overlying iliopsoas muscle. The main causes of iliopsoas bursitis include rheumatoid arthritis (RA), OA, trauma, total hip arthroplasty and overuse injury (Toohey *et al.* 1990). Iliopsoas bursitis and tendinitis are interrelated in the sense that inflammation of one will inevitably lead to inflammation of the other because of their close proximity.

CASE STUDY – RECOVERING FROM A TOTAL HIP REPLACEMENT (ARTHROPLASTY)

D is a yoga, Pilates and movement teacher with a professional dance background. She has had a total hip replacement of both of her hips.

1. Please share your experience of practicing yoga again after your surgery.

    Well I didn't practice yoga asana for about six weeks after surgery. But I did practice healing meditation and Yoga Nidra. I walked from day one and started practicing very basic Pilates after two weeks.

2. Were there certain movements that you needed to avoid during the rehabilitation process?

During the first six weeks I couldn't twist towards the operated hip. I couldn't bend the hip more than 90° with any movement. I couldn't lie on my side. I couldn't cross my legs. I did sit and stand tall and use my dumbbells for weight-lifting moves for arms and upper body. I stretched out with yoga poses like Eagle arms and Cow Face Pose. I also did a lot of ballet arms and kept a close eye on my posture when walking. I was able to get rid of one crutch within a week and the second within two weeks.

3. What advice would you give to a student who is rehabilitating from this surgery?

Be patient. Don't rush into lots of physical activity. I found that some people panic and think they need to do lots of exercises and training too soon, trying to get back to full strength before the deeper healing inside is done. They sometimes end up with complications. Healing meditation, visualization techniques, breathing/Pranayama are all great tools. I found these elements of the yoga practice so helpful for speeding up healing and recovery and getting through the whole process. I took it slow, never forced any movements and gradually over three to four months I had 50% of my yoga moves back and 80% movement back after a year! My energy levels shot up after the second hip was replaced. Constant pain can be so exhausting. My hypnosis techniques were very helpful with controlling pain. I had a spinal tap for the operation with a mild sedative. You recover from the anesthetic more quickly that way.

4. Has your range of movement been affected?

My left leg/hip is 100% perfect now. I can do all yoga poses that I had practiced before. My right hip/leg is at 80%. My right hip was the worst one and I had struggled with it for over ten years before surgery. I can't jump on my right leg or run leading with the right leg. I can't practice the splits anymore.

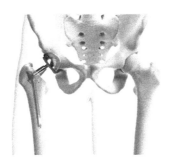

Total hip replacement

Key yoga asanas and how to adapt them

We will now explore some asanas that may present a challenge to students who are affected by the common injuries or conditions that we have discussed above and look at some of the ways that these can be adapted in order to make them more accessible.

Forward folds

In Seated Forward Fold (Paschimottanasana) it is helpful to raise the seat using a blanket, cushion or bolster. Keep the knees slightly bent and walk the hands forward along the thighs or the mat. For a longer hold a chair can be placed over the legs to support the upper body.

In Standing Forward Fold (Uttanasana) there is always the option to bend the knees slightly and place the hands on the thighs or on blocks placed in front. Half Standing Forward Fold (Ardha Uttanasana) can be practiced using a chair or a wall for support.

In Extended Triangle Pose (Utthita Trikonasana) a chair can be used as support for the lower arm so that the amount of flexion of the front hip can be more easily controlled.

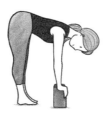

Standing Forward Fold

'Hip openers'

Easy Pose (Sukhasana) can be huge challenge for a student who is working with a hip condition or injury. Sitting up on blocks, blankets or a bolster is often really helpful here and it can feel really supportive to place a rolled-up blanket between the outer thighs and the mat. If in doubt, explore any other more comfortable seated position.

Some more accessible variations of Pigeon Pose (Eka Pada Rajaka-potasana) include Supine Pigeon Pose and Seated Pigeon Pose. In both variations the front foot can be stepped further forward so that less external rotation of the lifted hip is required in order to cross the lifted foot over the front thigh.

Warrior 1 (Virabhadrasana I) can be practiced with the front thigh resting on the support of a chair. A shorter stance can always be adopted with the feet placed hip-distance wide instead of the heels being placed in one line. Warrior 1 can also be practiced while sitting slightly diagonally on a chair. High Lunge is often a good alternative to this asana, particularly when lowering the back heel to the mat feels uncomfortable for the hips.

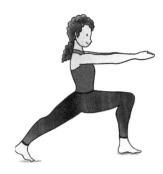

High Lunge

Garland Pose (Malasana) can be practiced sitting on a stack of wide yoga blocks to raise the seat. Goddess Pose (Utkata Konasana) can also be a more accessible alternative to this pose, particularly when practiced while sitting on the edge of a stable chair.

Asanas focusing on hip extension

Dancer Pose (Natarajasana) can be practiced using a strap to bind the raised foot as it lifts behind you. Using the support of a chair or wall in front of you or beside you can also be a great help. Dancer Pose can also be while sitting diagonally on a chair so that there is room to move the back hip into extension.

Bow Pose (Dhanurasana) can be practiced by slowly lifting one leg at a time, and a strap looped over the feet can be a great help.

Reclining Hero Pose (Supta Virasana) can be practiced by supporting the upper body with bolsters, stacked blocks or a chair.

Improving the overall health of the hip joint

This section addresses some effective ways in which we can all improve and maintain the health and functioning of our hips. It is intended to be a general guide for yoga practitioners and teachers and is not a replacement for the personal advice of a health professional.

Since the hip joint is so hugely impacted by the knee, the ankle and the foot, all of the exercises described in Chapters 1 and 2 will play an important role in the health and function of the hip joint.

Strengthening the hip musculature

A great exercise for the external rotators of the hip joint is the 'clam'.

1. Lie on your side with your hip bones and legs stacked.

2. Bend your knees to 90° so that your ankles and hips are roughly in one line along the length of your mat.

3. Gently brace your abdomen.

4. Place your top hand on the side of your top hip bone to keep it steady.

5. Keep your feet touching and slowly lift your top knee, moving from the hip joint.

6. Control the movement back so that your knees touch again.

7. After a few slow repetitions remove your top hand from your hip

bone but keep the pelvis in a fixed position as you move the hip. (We will explore the significance of isolating hip movement later in this section.)

8. Continue to build strength by tying a resistance band around the midsection of your thigh and repeating this exercise.

9. Repeat the exercises on the other side.

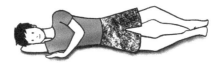

The 'clam'

For the internal rotators, 'inverse clam' is an accessible exercise for most people.

1. Start in the position described above.

2. Keep your knees touching or gently hug a blanket between your knees.

3. Widen the top ankle away from the bottom ankle.

4. Slowly lower back down and after a few repetitions repeat this on the other side.

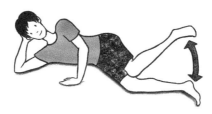

The 'inverse clam'

Here is another great exercise for focusing on internal hip rotation.

1. Lie on your back with your knees bent and feet stepped out to the sides of your mat.

2. Place your hands onto the front of your hip bones to steady your pelvis.

3. Keep your left leg fixed in this position.

4. Spread across your right foot and slowly lower your right knee down towards the midline.

5. Raise your knee back and repeat this a few times.

6. Once you have completed both sides, remove your hands from your pelvis.

7. Repeat the exercise and keep the pelvis in a fixed position without the help of your hands.

8. To increase the load in this exercise it can be repeated while sitting on blocks, eventually working up to a Garland Pose (Malasana) variation.

For the hip extensors we are going to focus on Bridge Pose (Setu Bandha Sarvangasana) variations.

1. Lie on your back with your knees bent and ankles roughly under your knees.

2. Press your feet down into the mat and slowly raise your pelvis up off the mat.

3. After a couple of breaths slowly lower your pelvis back.

4. Now step your feet a couple of inches further away from your pelvis and repeat the exercise.

5. An option here is to pivot on your heels as you lift.

6. Over time you can work towards stepping your feet further and further away from your pelvis.

7. You can also work on holding the position for longer.

8. To increase the load, once you have lifted your pelvis begin to lift one foot or heel off the ground at a time.

Another challenging variation here is to place your feet on a blanket and smooth floor instead of your mat. Slowly draw your feet or heels away from your pelvis and then back towards your pelvis.

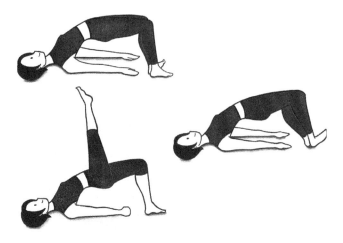

Extended Bridge Pose and variations

For the hip abductors we will adopt a similar position as the set up for 'clam'.

1. Lie on your side with your hip bones and legs stacked.

2. This time straighten your top leg along the length of the mat.

3. Place your top hand onto your top hip bone and brace your abdomen.

4. Slowly lift your top foot, focusing the movement at the hip joint.

5. Lower your leg back down.

6. After a couple of repetitions repeat this with the other leg.

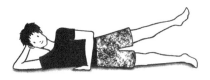

Lateral leg raise

To increase the load, come to standing position and strap a resistance band around your ankles. Slowly step the right foot to the right, away from the left foot, against the resistance of the band. Step the left foot in to meet the right foot and repeat this a few times. Then start by leading with the left foot.

For the hip adductors we will need a blanket and a smooth floor.

1. Start on the floor on your hands and knees with your knees wide and placed on the blanket.

2. Slowly draw your knees towards each other and then apart again to repeat the exercise.

To add load to this exercise you can repeat it in a Saddle Pose position.

1. Have your big toes touching, your knees wide and placed on the blanket, and sit back on your heels using whatever support you need.

2. Slowly draw your knees towards each other and then apart again to repeat the exercise.

3. An additional variation involves kneeling on the blanket with your knees wide and once again drawing your knees towards each other.

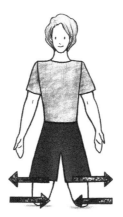

Kneeling adduction

This exercise is for the hip flexors.

1. Start by standing with one foot lifted in front of you.

2. Rest this foot on a step or a low chair.

3. Brace your abdomen and slowly lift your raised foot up off the support.

4. Hold this position for a couple of breaths before lowering your foot back down.

5. Repeat this with your other leg.

6. To add load to this exercise you can resist the movement by pressing down on your thigh with your hand.

This exercise strengthens the hip flexors in a seated position.

1. In Staff Pose (Dandasana) place a block to the outside of your right foot.

2. Brace your abdomen and keep your right leg straight.

3. Slowly lift your right foot up and over the block and then back to its original position.

4. Repeat this a few times with the option of increasing the height of the block.

5. Repeat this exercise on the right side.

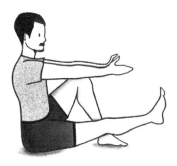

Hip flexor strengthening

Isolating hip movements from spinal movements

Learning to isolate hip movements from lumbar spine movements is an important skill that helps to develop proprioceptive awareness and can also improve hip mobility. Let's explore what I mean by this in Supine Pigeon Pose. When a student attempts to draw their top femur towards their torso they often tilt their pelvis posteriorly so that their sitz bones lift. The movement that takes place mainly comes from flexing their lumbar spine instead of flexing their hip. Flexing the spine isn't bad here but the intention might have been to flex the hip joint instead. So, to isolate the movement at the hip joint, the student can keep drawing their sitz bones down as they draw the femur back. A similar situation can arise in One-Legged Downward Dog Pose (Eka Pada Adho Mukha Svanasana). As the student lifts their leg high behind themselves, they allow their lower ribs to lift towards their mat. A significant amount of the movement is coming from their lumbar and thoracic spine extending rather than their hip joint extending. Again, this isn't necessarily problematic, but the student is missing out on an opportunity to specifically work on developing their hip extension range of movement. By keeping their front lower ribs drawing towards their back lower ribs as they lift their leg, the movement takes place predominantly at their hip joint.

IS FOAM ROLLING EFFECTIVE?

There is widespread belief that foam rolling helps to break down 'fascial adhesions' in areas such as the ITB. Let's first look at some of the research that has been done on the potential benefits of foam rolling and then explore the possible underlying mechanisms.

Cheatham *et al.* (2015) conducted a systematic review of literature that looked at the effects of foam rolling on joint range of movement, muscle recovery and performance. They report that foam rolling may have short-term effects of increasing joint range of motion without decreasing muscle performance. The results also indicate a reduction in perceived pain after an intense bout of exercise. The review states that there currently is no consensus on the optimal foam rolling intervention (treatment time, pressure and cadence).

Wiewelhove *et al.* (2019) conducted a meta-analysis of literature that looked at the effects of foam rolling on performance and recovery. They report that the effects of foam rolling on performance and recovery are rather minor and partly negligible, but can be relevant in some cases, for example to increase sprint performance and flexibility or to reduce muscle pain sensation. They conclude that the evidence seems to justify the widespread use of foam rolling as a warm-up activity rather than a recovery tool.

While it is clear that foam rolling has some benefits for some people, it is important to mention that few studies have examined the potential underlying mechanisms. The effects of foam rolling have been attributed to mechanical, neurological, physiological and psychophysiological parameters but these are theorized and not based on strong evidence. These mechanisms include: reduction in tissue adhesion and scar tissue; altered tissue stiffness; the potentiation of analgesic effects and muscular recovery by mediating pain-modulatory systems; increased blood flow and parasympathetic circulation, as well as inflammatory responses and associated trigger-point breakdown; and improved perceptions of wellbeing and recovery due to the increase of plasma endorphins, decreased arousal level, an activation of the parasympathetic response and/or the placebo effect.

So, in summary, if you are currently using a foam roller and feel the benefit from it then keep it up. But if you are not using a foam roller and feel like you're missing out, don't lose any sleep over it.

Chapter 4

THE PELVIS

The anatomy of the pelvis

The two hip bones join with the sacrum and the coccyx to form the bowl-shaped pelvis (Latin for 'basin'). The bones of the pelvis are strongly united to each other to form a largely immobile, weight-bearing structure. The pelvis is the area where the lower limbs attach to the axial skeleton through the sacroiliac (SI) joints and therefore plays important roles in movement. The bony pelvis comes together to provide support for the pelvic muscles and connective tissues, which, in turn, provide attachments and support for the pelvic organs.

Because of the important role of the pelvis in pregnancy and childbirth, it is one of the bony elements of the human body that differs most between sexes. As always, there is also wide variation between different members of the same sex. A study by Fischer and Mitteroecker (2017) reported that while overall pelvic size is similar in both sexes, the shape of the pelvis differs considerably. They found that the distributions of male and female pelvis shape showed only very little overlap, allowing for a reliable sex identification (98% correctly classified individuals). Their analysis showed that pelvis size and shape are similarly associated with stature in both sexes.

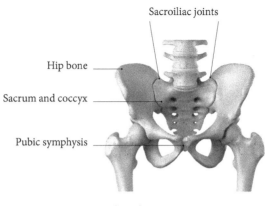

Sacroiliac joints

Hip bone

Sacrum and coccyx

Pubic symphysis

The pelvis

The bony architecture of the hip bones

In the immature skeleton the hip bone is made up of three separate bones: the ilium, the ischium and the pubis. Fusion of these three bones starts to occur around the age of 14–16 years and is usually complete by the age of 23 (Moore 1992). The cup-shaped acetabulum, or hip socket, is formed at the area where these three bones meet.

The curved superior margin of the ilium is the iliac crest. You can feel the iliac crest on both sides of the pelvis by placing your hands on your waist and pressing down slightly. The rounded, anterior termination of the iliac crest is the anterior superior iliac spine (ASIS) which can be felt at the anterolateral pelvis. Inferior to the ASIS is a rounded protuberance called the anterior inferior iliac spine (AIIS). Both of these iliac spines serve as attachment points for muscles of the thigh. Posteriorly, the iliac crest curves downward to terminate as the posterior superior iliac spine (PSIS). Muscles and ligaments surround but do not cover this bony landmark and often a depression or dimple can be seen on the skin of this region on the lower back. More inferiorly is the posterior inferior iliac spine (PIIS). Both the PSIS and the PIIS serve as attachment points for the muscles and very strong ligaments that support the SI joint.

The main bony landmarks on the ischium are the ischial tuberosities. They serve as the attachment for the posterior thigh muscles and also carry the weight of the body when we are sitting. They are often referred to as the 'sitting bones' or 'sitz bones' (from the German verb 'sitzen' meaning 'to sit').

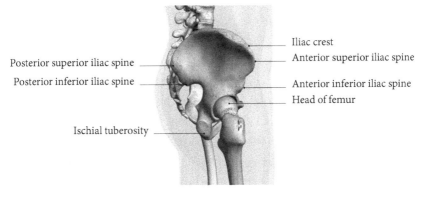

Lateral view of the pelvis

INTELLIGENT MOVEMENT PRINCIPLE – OUR BODY IS NOT SYMMETRICAL AND NEVER WILL BE

No two pelvises are exactly the same shape or size and no pelvis is symmetrical in any plane. So, what might look or feel like a 'neutral' pelvis for one person will look and feel different for the next person. This makes the concepts of squaring the hip bones or keeping the pelvis level both challenging and arbitrary. How can we clearly define what an anteriorly tilted pelvis is if we all have such unique structures in the first place?

Instead of being fixated with the shape of an asana or even with our own standing posture, it is a great idea to spend more time getting to know our unique bodies, exploring both subtle and gross movements and focusing more on the experience of practicing yoga asanas rather than on their form. A wonderful statement that I have been unable to find the original source of is: Use yoga asanas to get into the body and not the body to get into yoga asanas.

The sacrum

The sacrum (Latin for sacred) is a large triangular bone originating from separate vertebra that fuse along with the intervening intervertebral discs. One of the functions of the sacrum is to transmit the weight of the body to the hip bones.

Anatomical variations occur frequently in this region, making the sacrum the most variable section of the spine (Esses and Botsford 1997). While most sacra have five fused vertebrae, the number of fused vertebrae can vary from four to seven. The variations consist of the sacralization of the L5 vertebra (i.e., L5 fuses with S1 to become part of the sacrum), the lumbarization of the S1 vertebra (i.e., S1 remains unfused to S2 and acts as part of the lumbar section) or the incorporation of the first piece of the coccyx to the sacrum (Singh, Ajita and Singh 2015).

The sacrum articulates with four bones: the most inferior lumbar vertebra above via a disc space and facet joint complex, the coccyx below with a ligamentous attachment and occasional bone union, and on either side with the ilium via the SI joint.

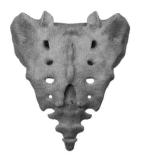

Posterior view of sacrum and coccyx

The SI joints

The SI joint is the largest axial joint in the body and is formed by the crescent-shaped articulation between the medial surface of the ilium and the lateral surface of the sacrum. The articulating surface of the sacrum is slightly concave to fit the convex surface of the ilium.

There is wide variability in the size, shape and surface contour of the adult SI joint. The same individual may even have large disparities between their right and left SI joint (Ruch 1997). Age-related changes in the SI joint begin at puberty and continue throughout life.

Its superior and posterior region forms a fibrous joint in which the joint surfaces are bound by interosseous ligaments. A cartilaginous zone extends through the two lower thirds of the anterior zone, which in reality has the structure of a symphysis with hyaline cartilage firmly bound to the adjacent bone by fibrous tissue. Only the anterior third forms a true synovial joint (García Díez *et al.* 2009).

With this complex arrangement the SI joints are designed primarily for stability. Their functions include the transmission and dissipation of loads from the axial spine into the lower limbs and facilitating childbirth. During pregnancy, the SI joint's fibrous apparatus loosens under the influence of the hormone relaxin, resulting in an increase in SI joint mobility.

The interlocking symmetrical grooves and ridges of the SI joint articular surfaces contribute to the highest amount of friction of any moveable joint in the human body. The keystone-like bony anatomy of the sacrum further contributes to stability within the pelvic ring. The sacrum is wider superiorly than inferiorly and also wider anteriorly than posteriorly, permitting the sacrum to become 'wedged' into the ilia within the pelvic ring. These properties are believed to enhance the stability of the joint against shearing from vertical compression (e.g., gravity) and anteriorly directed forces on the spine (Vleeming *et al.* 2012).

SI joint stability is also provided by the strongest ligament system in the body. This includes the anterior and posterior sacroiliac ligaments, the sacrospinous ligament running from the sacrum to the ischial spine, the sacrotuberous ligament running from the sacrum to the ischial tuberosity and the interosseous ligament which is the strongest ligament in the body. The interosseous ligament lies deep to the posterior ligament and consists of a series of short, strong fibers forming the major connection between the sacrum and the ilium. All of these ligaments help to support and immobilize the sacrum as it carries the weight of the body.

The SI joint is additionally supported by a network of muscles that helps to deliver regional muscular forces to the pelvic bones. Some of these muscles, such as the gluteus maximus, piriformis, biceps femoris and the lower lumbar multifidi and erector spinae, are functionally connected to SI joint ligaments.

The SI joint rotates about all three axes, although the movements are very small and difficult to measure. In a study by Egund *et al.* (1978) the authors found the maximal rotations and translations of the SI joints in their subjects to be 2.0° and 2.0 mm, respectively. A larger study by Jacob and Kissling (1995) found similarly small limits on rotation (1.7°) and translation (0.7 mm). Kibsgård *et al.* (2014) reported that movement in the SI joint during a single-leg stance is small and almost undetectable.

Two of the main movements of the SI joint are nutation and counternutation. Nutation (forward nodding) occurs as the sacrum moves anteriorly and inferiorly while the coccyx moves posteriorly relative to the ilium. This movement causes the ischial tuberosities to subtly widen apart and the ASISs to subtly narrow towards each other. Counternutation (backward nodding) occurs as the sacrum moves posteriorly and superiorly while the coccyx moves anteriorly relative to the ilium. This movement causes the ischial tuberosities to subtly narrow towards each and the ASISs to subtly widen apart. These changes in the shape of the pelvis are very important during childbirth.

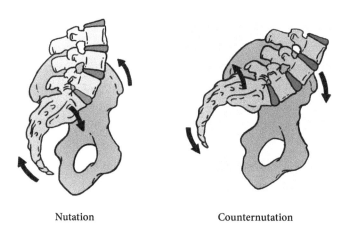

Nutation   Counternutation

Although muscular influence on movement of the SI joint has long been disputed, the erector spinae and multifidi muscles are thought to assist in pulling the sacrum into nutation (Vleeming *et al.* 2012). We will explore these muscles in the next chapter. Steinke *et al.* (2010) suggested that nutation tightens most of the SI joint ligaments, thereby preparing the pelvis for increased loading. During pelvic-floor contraction the coccyx moves forward and up towards the pubic symphysis (Raizada and Mittal 2008). This action counternutates the SI joint.

Mitchell and Pruzzo (1971) demonstrated that the sacrum moves into nutation on exhalation and counternutation on inhalation. Based on research by Frymann (1971), craniosacral therapy techniques are based on the belief that movement of cerebral spinal fluid is coordinated with reciprocating movement of the cranium and sacrum. There is still considerable controversy within the research community about whether this mechanism actually exists independently of respiration and cardiac rhythms.

The coccyx

The word coccyx is derived from the Greek word for the beak of a cuckoo bird. Often referred to as the tailbone, the coccyx articulates with the inferior end of the sacrum via the sacrococcygeal (SC) joint. The joint is reinforced by anterior, posterior and lateral SC ligaments (Gray *et al.* 2005).

Despite its small size, the coccyx has several important functions including serving as the insertion site for multiple muscles, ligaments and tendons. The coccyx also provides positional support to the anus (Smallwood Lirette *et al.* 2014) and joins the ischial tuberosities to form a tripod that provides weight-bearing support when we sit.

The normal adult coccyx comprises between three and five vertebrae, with four being present in most individuals. A study by Woon *et al.* (2013) reported that coccyges had either three (13%), four (76%) or five vertebrae (11%) and there was no evidence for an association with gender. They found that the sacrococcygeal joint was fused in 57% of coccyges, the first intercoccygeal joint in 17%, the second in 61%, the third in 89% of coccyges with four vertebrae, and the fourth in all coccyges with five vertebrae. Fusion of all sacrococcygeal and intercoccygeal joints was relatively rare (3% in this study).

During pelvic-floor contraction the coccyx moves forward and up towards the pubic symphysis (Raizada and Mittal 2008) and this action counternutates the SI joints.

The pubic symphysis

The pubic symphysis is a unique joint consisting of a fibrocartilaginous disc sandwiched between the articular surfaces of the pubic bones. Four ligaments reinforce the joint, which resists tensile, shearing and compressive forces and is capable of a small amount of multidirectional movement in most adults (up to 2 mm shift and 1° rotation). During pregnancy, circulating hormones such as relaxin induce resorption of the symphyseal margins and structural changes in the fibrocartilaginous disc, significantly increasing the width and mobility of the pubic symphysis (Becker, Woodley and Stringer 2010).

The pelvic-floor musculature

While there is no consensus amongst the scientific literature regarding the exact definition of the 'pelvic floor', we will explore this complex musculature in terms of three layers: the muscular pelvic diaphragm, the puborectalis and the urogenital diaphragm.

The deep pelvic-floor muscles consist of pubococcygeus and iliococcygeus (which are often grouped together to be called levator ani) and coccygeus. These three muscles can be thought of as the muscular pelvic diaphragm. The muscular pelvic diaphragm changes in shape from a basin to a dome during contraction, providing support for the pelvic organs (Raizada and Mittal 2008). This layer of muscles is also involved during forced expiration. Two of the deep external hip rotators can also be found in this region. Piriformis is part of the pelvic sidewall and is located posteriorly and lateral to coccygeus. Obturator internus has an intimate anatomical relationship to levator ani.

Puborectalis muscle is located in between the superficial and deep muscle layers and provides the constrictor function to the anal canal, vagina and urethra (Raizada and Mittal 2008).

The urogenital diaphragm is a strong, muscular membrane that occupies the area between the pubic symphysis and ischial tuberosities. The urogenital diaphragm is superficial and inferior to the muscular pelvic diaphragm and puborectalis. It comprises of the urethral sphincter, the external anal sphincter and the urogenital triangle (including the superficial transverse perineal muscle).

In yoga the pelvic-floor region can be thought of as the anatomical reference point for mula bandha, which is an energetic seal or lock.

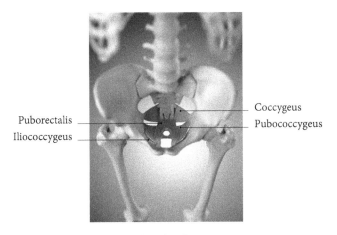

Puborectalis

Iliococcygeus

Coccygeus

Pubococcygeus

The pelvic floor

TO TUCK OR NOT TO TUCK?

The topic of whether we should tuck the tailbone or not in our yoga practice is a popular and controversial one. It is important to note that these terms have different meanings to different people. Tucking can refer to posteriorly tilting the pelvis or to counternutating the SI joints. Untucking can refer to anteriorly tilting the pelvis or nutating the SI joints. Both the anterior and posterior tilt of the pelvis come from the lumbar spine and/or the hip joints.

All of these are natural movements and none of them are inherently right or wrong. Whether you choose to tuck or untuck your tailbone is going to depend on your unique anatomy, your typical sitting and standing posture and what your intent is for a particular asana.

If you tend to round your lower back when you stand so that you have a shallow lumbar curve you can try untucking your tailbone by spreading your sitting bones as you roll your upper, inner thighs back. Internally rotating your hip joints will cause your SI joints to subtly nutate and allow you to create a deeper lumbar curve.

If you lean more towards a deeper curve in your lumbar spine you can try tucking your tailbone by drawing your sitting bones closer as you roll your upper, inner thighs forward. Externally rotating your hip joints will cause your SI joints to subtly counternutate and allow you to create a shallower lumbar curve.

Most of us would probably benefit from regularly tucking and untucking our tailbones in a controlled way. After all, movement is medicine.

Common pelvic injuries and conditions

In this section we will explore some of the most common pelvic injuries and conditions that affect our population.

Pelvic-floor dysfunction (PFD)

PFD is a term that refers to a broad range of clinical scenarios, including urinary and anal incontinence, overactive bladder and pelvic organ prolapse, as well as sexual disorders.

Healthy pelvic-floor muscles are able to voluntarily and involuntarily contract and relax.

The muscles can become overactive (they do not relax or may even contract when relaxation is functionally needed), underactive (they cannot voluntarily contract when this is appropriate) or non-functioning (there is no action at all).

In developing countries, the prevalence of pelvic organ prolapses, urinary incontinence and anal incontinence is 19.7%, 28.7% and 6.9%, respectively (Bozkurt, Yumru and Şahin 2014). The prevalence increases significantly with age. By age 80, 11% of women have undergone surgery for pelvic-organ prolapse or urinary incontinence (Handa *et al.* 2003).

The etiology of PFD is unknown but probably multifactorial. PFD is often associated with childbirth: many studies in the literature define traumatic birth, usage of forceps, length of the second stage of delivery and sphincter damage as modifiable risk factors for PFD (Bozkurt *et al.* 2014). The loss of strength of connective tissues may induce PFD formation as a result of hormonal changes, particularly estrogen deficiency related to advancing age and duration of postmenopausal state.

SI dysfunction

The SI joint has long been implicated as a source of low back and lower extremity pain. There are no definite historical, physical or radiological features that can definitively establish a diagnosis of SI joint pain. Presently, small-volume diagnostic nerve blocks remain the most commonly used method for diagnosing this disorder, although their validity remains unproven.

It is important to note that the exact cause of SI pain and dysfunction is not fully understood and is likely to be multifactorial. Palsson *et al.* (2019) suggested that clinicians should address unhelpful beliefs about structural fragility instead of reinforcing these.

The three broad categories of SI joint pain are: pregnancy-related SI joint pain, specific pathology of the SI joint (e.g., fracture) and SI joint-related pain of other origin.

In all SI joints, starting around 50 years of age, some sort of degeneration is seen, and these changes are more profuse in women than in men of the same age, progressing faster in women who have given birth compared to those who have not (García Díez *et al.* 2009). Compared to the lumbar spine, the SI joints can withstand a much greater medially directed force but only half the torsion and one-twentieth of the axial compression load (Dreyfuss, Cole and Pauza 2004). These last two motions may preferentially strain and injure the weaker anterior joint capsule of the SI joint (Dreyfuss *et al.* 1995). Pregnancy can result in SI joint pain by virtue of weight gain, exaggerated lordotic posture, third-trimester hormone-induced ligamentous relaxation and the pelvic trauma associated with childbirth.

Symphysis pubis dysfunction (SPD)

SPD is a relatively common but poorly understood condition affecting athletes and patients with traumatic pelvic injuries, but mainly pregnant women. Symptoms of SPD include shooting pain in the symphysis pubis, radiating pain into the lower abdomen, back, groin, perineum, thigh and/ or leg, and pain on movement, especially walking, unilateral weight-bearing or hip abduction.

The incidence of pelvic pain in pregnancy has been reported as between 48% and 71%, and pubic symphysis dysfunction has been reported in 31.7% of pregnant women (Howell 2012). Studies on the relationship between widening of the pubic symphysis, symphyseal symptoms and circulating concentrations of relaxin have yielded conflicting results (Becker *et al.* 2010).

Coccydynia

Coccydynia presents as debilitating pain in the coccygeal region, exacerbated by sitting, standing and/or walking. It is a common condition that is often self-limited (Smallwood Lirette *et al.* 2014). The prevalence of coccydynia is four times higher in women than men. Most cases are considered to arise from sacrococcygeal or intercoccygeal joint instability, which is often traumatic in origin. Trauma may be acute from a fall or during childbirth, or chronic and repetitive, when obesity may be a predisposing factor. However, in one-third of cases the cause is unknown (Karadimas, Trypsiannis and Giannoudis 2011).

Ankylosing spondylitis (AS)

AS is a persistent inflammatory arthritis within a family of related disorders including psoriatic arthritis and inflammatory bowel disease. It has a gradual onset and largely affects the axial skeleton. The hallmark feature of ankylosing spondylitis is the involvement of the SI joints during the progression of the disease. In its extreme form AS can lead to the bony fusion of vertebral joints and is an uncommon but well-established cause of persistent back pain.

Paget's disease of bone (PDB)

PDB is characterized by focal bone lesions in which there is increased bone resorption coupled with increased and disorganized new bone formation. The most common sites are the pelvis, spine, femur, skull and tibia. Many patients are asymptomatic, and a common mode of presentation is with an abnormal blood test or an abnormal radiograph (Ralston 2013).

The most common complaint in patients who come to medical attention is bone pain. Other common complications include pathological fractures, bone deformity, deafness (when the base of the skull is involved), secondary osteoarthritis and nerve compression syndromes (van Staa *et al.* 2002).

PDB is estimated to affect about 1–2% of people above the age of 55. A family history is found in approximately 15% of cases. PDB is common in Europe with the UK having the highest prevalence of PDB in the world. One of the most important risk factors for developing PDB is increasing age; the disease is rare below the age of 50 years, but the prevalence doubles each decade thereafter to affect up to 8% of men and 5% of women by the age of 80 in the UK (van Staa *et al.* 2002).

Key yoga asanas and how to adapt them

We will now explore some asanas that may present a challenge to students who are affected by the common injuries or conditions that we have discussed above and look at some of the ways that these can be adapted in order to make them more accessible.

Twists

In supine twists it a good idea to stabilize the pelvis and move the upper body instead of stabilizing the upper body and moving the pelvis. Start by lying on your side with your hip bones stacked and a blanket between your thighs. Begin to roll your top shoulder back towards the floor. If your shoulder and arm do not comfortably rest on the floor they can be supported with a blanket, cushion or bolster. Another option is to straighten your bottom leg in line with your spine and rest your top knee and lower leg onto a bolster.

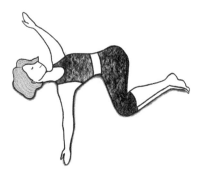

Supine twist

A helpful principle in twists is to allow your pelvis to move in the direction of the main force in the asana. In a seated twist the main force will be the rotation of your spine. So, instead of trying to fix the base of your pelvis to the mat, allow your pelvis to subtly move in the direction of the twist. In a standing asana such as Warrior 2 (Virabhadrasana II) the main force will be the external rotation of your front hip joint. Instead of trying to 'square' your pelvis to the side, allow your pelvis to subtly turn in the direction of your front thigh.

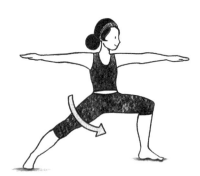

The pelvis subtly moving in the direction of the front thigh in Warrior 2

In twists it is helpful to focus on mobility over flexibility (we will discuss this principle in greater detail in Chapter 10). It can be easy to rely on external force to move us into twists and to hold us in position, but we therefore miss the opportunity to use our core musculature to do the work and risk applying too much force to our pelvis and lumbar spine. In seated twists, and in standing twists such as Revolved Chair (Parivrtta Utkatasana), slowly rotate your spine and upper body without using your opposite arm as a lever. Once you are in position you can rest your opposite arm against your leg to help maintain the natural curves of your spine but ideally you should be able to stay in position if you release your arm.

Forward folds

Asanas such as Head-to-Knee Pose (Janu Sirsasana), Bound Angle Pose (Baddha Konasana) and Wide-Angle Seated Forward Bend (Upavistha Konasana) can prove to be particularly challenging for students who are working with pelvic injuries and conditions.

In Head-to-Knee Pose (Janu Sirsasana), be sure that your pelvis tilts forward with your spine. It can help to sit on a foam block or folded blanket. Focus on bringing the bent-knee side of the pelvis forward and you may want to practice the pose with your foot touching the opposite knee instead of the inner thigh. The upper body can be supported with bolsters and foam blocks.

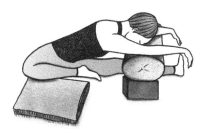

Head-to-Knee Pose

In Bound Angle Pose (Baddha Konasana) and Wide-Angle Seated Forward Bend (Upavistha Konasana) raising your seat with a foam block, cushion or folded blanket is a good start.

A rolled-up blanket under the outer thighs can be a great support in Bound Angle Pose, particularly for a restorative version of the asana where one stays in the position for longer. Move slowly and mindfully while imagining that you are gently hugging your pelvis. In Wide-Angle

Seated Forward Bend bring your legs closer together than usual and rest your arms and forehead on a chair or stack of foam blocks in front of you.

Improving the overall health of the pelvis

This section addresses some effective ways in which we can all improve and maintain the health and functioning of our pelvis. It is intended to be a general guide for yoga practitioners and teachers and is not a replacement for the personal advice of a health professional.

Pelvic-floor muscle (PFM) training

Kegel (1948) is credited with introducing PFM training as an effective therapy for urinary incontinence in women. The theoretical rationale for intensive strength training of the PFM is that strength training may build up the structural support of the pelvis by elevating the levator plate to a permanent higher location inside the pelvis and by enhancing hypertrophy and stiffness of the PFM and connective tissue.

A literature review by Bø (2012) reported that PFM training has support from several high-quality studies as treatment for urinary incontinence and pelvic organ prolapse. The studies found that PFM training has no known serious adverse effects and suggested that it should therefore be offered as first-line treatment for these conditions. They stated that there is also some evidence to support an effect on sexual function.

Therapy is ideally provided by a physical therapist with training in pelvic-floor dysfunction. The specific therapy used is guided by symptoms and usually includes strategies to optimize lumbopelvic and spinal function and to improve bowel, bladder and sexual function.

Core exercises

Bø (2004) stated that contractions of other large muscle groups such as the gluteal muscles, hip adductors and abdominals result in a simultaneous contraction, or 'co-contraction', of the pelvic-floor muscles. However, unlike the PFM, these other muscle groups are not in an anatomical position to act as a structural support to prevent bladder neck and urethral descent.

Training the PFM indirectly through training the transverse abdominis muscles is based on results from small experimental studies and does not seem to have any support in the general exercise science literature.

A small study by Richardson *et al.* (2002) reported that contraction of the transversus abdominis significantly decreases the laxity of the sacroiliac joint. This decrease in laxity is larger than that caused by a bracing action using all the lateral abdominal muscles.

We will discuss the core musculature and core exercises in greater detail in the next chapter.

Proprioceptive training

Broadly defined, proprioception can be thought of as awareness of the body and has several distinct properties: passive motion sense, active motion sense, limb position sense and the sense of heaviness. Proprioceptive training can therefore be thought of as an intervention that targets the improvement of proprioceptive function and therefore the improvement of sensorimotor function (Aman *et al.* 2015).

Let's look at a simple proprioception exercise for the pelvis.

1. Lie on your back with your knees bent and feet flat.

2. Slowly begin to tilt your pelvis back and forward. This can be thought of as Supine Cat-Cow Pose (Chakravakasana).

3. Start to become aware of how you are controlling these movements.

4. The mat and floor will help to provide feedback so that you can become more aware of the positions of your pelvis.

5. Now begin to roll your pelvis clockwise, tilting it forward, to the right, backwards and to the left.

6. Initiate the movements by pressing your feet down and then see if you can roll your pelvis without pressing through your feet.

7. After a few repetitions, repeat this in the opposite direction.

We can now explore some further Cat-Cow Pose variations.

1. Start with the classic version on your hands and knees.

2. Move as slowly as you can through the gentle backbending and forward-folding sequence.

3. Again, start to become more aware of how you are actually making these subtle movements happen.

4. Begin to make pelvic circles in one direction and then the opposite direction, controlling each subtle movement.

5. Stay within pain-free range.

6. Come back to a neutral position on your hands and knees.

7. Stabilize your upper spine and attempt to only move your lower spine and pelvis as you practice Cat-Cow Pose again. This can take time and patience.

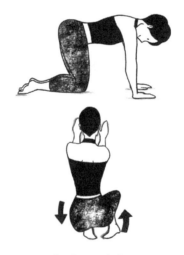

Cat-Cow variation

Back in your neutral position on your hands and knees, brace your abdomen and slowly lift your knees a couple of inches off the mat, keeping your pelvis stabilized. Hold this position for a couple of breaths before slowly lowering your knees back to the floor. Repeat this a couple of times, eventually increasing the length of the hold.

The exercises in the previous chapter that looked at isolating hip movements from pelvic movements will also help here, particularly the 'clam'.

1. Lie on your side with your hip bones and legs stacked.

2. Gently brace your abdomen.

3. Bend your knees to 90° so that your ankles and hips are roughly in one line along the length of your mat.

4. Place your top hand on the side of your top hip bone to keep it steady.

5. Keep your feet touching and slowly lift your top knee, moving from the hip joint.

6. Control the movement back so that your knees touch again.

7. After a few slow repetitions remove your top hand from your hip bone but keep the pelvis in a fixed position as you move only from the hip joint.

Part 2

THE SPINE
AND TRUNK

A free online class incorporating most of the practices
described in this part can be found at https://lddy.no/pat6.

—— Chapter 5 ——

THE VERTEBRAL COLUMN

An overview of spinal anatomy

The vertebral column, also known as our spine or backbone, is a multi-articular, segmented structure that is typically made up of 33 vertebrae along with many ligaments, muscles and intervertebral discs. As we have already discussed regarding the sacrum and coccyx, the number of vertebrae can vary between individuals. The vertebral column is separated into five main sections: the cervical spine, the thoracic spine, the lumbar spine, the sacrum and the coccyx. Within these sections, individual vertebrae are designated by letter (L for lumbar, T for thoracic, C for cervical and S for sacral) and identified by number from superior to inferior (e.g., the most superior thoracic vertebra is designated T1).

When viewed from the side, the sections are characteristically curved: cervical lordosis (concave); thoracic kyphosis (convex); lumbar lordosis (concave); and sacral kyphosis (convex). In the fetus the vertebral column is completely kyphotic ('C' shaped) and after birth the secondary curves develop: first in the cervical region when the child holds up its head, and then in the lumbar region when the legs start weight-bearing.

The structures that form the vertebral column must be rigid enough to support the trunk and the limbs, strong enough to protect the spinal cord and anchor the deep spinal muscles, and yet sufficiently flexible to allow for movement of the head and trunk in multiple directions. The curves of the spine make the structure particularly stable, allowing for the distribution of body weight and the absorption of shock, helping with balance and facilitating movement. The vertebrae also serve as a site for hemopoiesis, the production of blood cells and platelets.

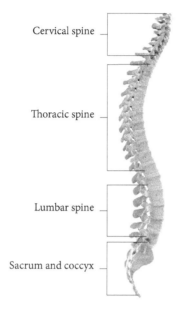

Cervical spine

Thoracic spine

Lumbar spine

Sacrum and coccyx

The vertebral column

Vertebral structure

Each vertebra consists of two main parts: the anterior body and the posterior vertebral arch.

The space between the body and the arch is the vertebral foramen. Each vertebra therefore forms a segment of the vertebral canal passing down the vertebral column, in which the spinal cord travels.

The vertebral body is the thick oval segment of bone forming the front of the vertebra. The cavity of the vertebral body consists of cancellous bone tissue and is encircled by a protective layer of compact bone. On the superior and inferior surface of each vertebral body are cartilaginous endplates which form the junction between the relatively hard and rigid vertebrae and the soft, flexible tissue of the intervertebral disc. The endplates are elegantly structured to enable the effective transmission of load.

The pedicle is the short segment of the arch close to the vertebral body. Its superior and inferior surfaces are notched for the spinal nerves that emerge from the spinal cord to innervate corresponding body segments. These nerves pass through the gaps between adjacent articulating vertebrae, which are called intervertebral foramina.

The arch of the vertebra has a posterior spinous process and two transverse processes which are attachment points for the many deep ligaments and muscles of the spine.

Successive vertebrae articulate directly with one another across small synovial joints. All moveable vertebrae have two superior and two inferior articular facets located on the vertebral arch. These four facets are lined with hyaline cartilage and control movement between adjacent vertebrae.

The shape and size of each vertebra is subtly different from its neighbor as we travel up the vertebral column. It is the orientation of the facet joints, along with the shape of the vertebral body and the shape and angle of the spinous process and the transverse processes, that determines the range of movement of each segment.

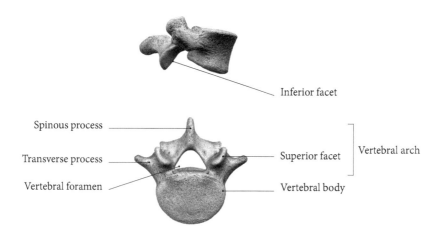

Vertebral structure from a lateral (top image) and superior (lower image) view

Spinal ligaments

Several ligaments connect the vertebrae together and, along with the deep spinal muscles, control and limit vertebral column movement.

There are three ligaments that run the length of the spinal column:

the anterior longitudinal ligament is attached to the front of the vertebral bodies and limits extension of the spine; the posterior longitudinal ligament is attached to the back of the vertebral bodies and limits flexion; the supraspinous ligament runs along the tips of the spinous processes and limits flexion.

The ligamentum flavum is composed of a series of strong, paired ligaments that span the space between the vertebral arches. Each component stretches laterally, joining the facet joint capsule.

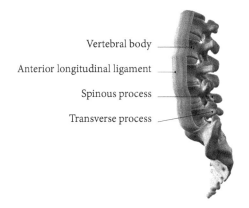

Vertebral body

Anterior longitudinal ligament

Spinous process

Transverse process

Anterolateral view of the anterior longitudinal ligament

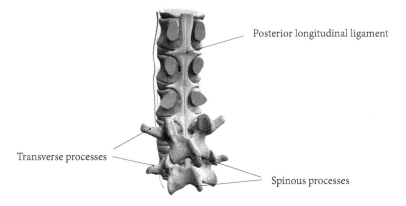

Posterior longitudinal ligament

Transverse processes

Spinous processes

Posterior longitudinal ligament with some of the vertebral arches removed

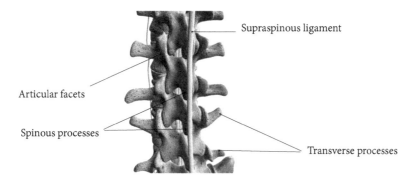

Supraspinous ligament

Articular facets

Spinous processes

Transverse processes

Supraspinous ligament

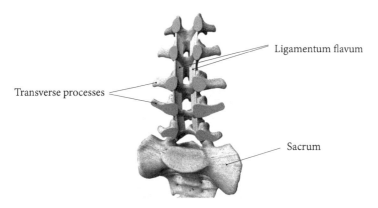

Ligamentum flavum

Transverse processes

Sacrum

Anterior view of the ligamentum flavum with the vertebral bodies removed

Intervertebral discs

The intervertebral disc is a cartilaginous and articulating structure between the vertebral bodies. Intervertebral discs have the dual role of providing the primary support for the vertebral column while possessing enough elasticity to permit the required mobility of the spine. The discs account for 25–30% of the overall height of the spine. We are tallest first thing in the morning when the discs are their most plump, and we slowly become shorter during the day as the discs subtly flatten under our body weight (Botsford, Esses and Ogilvie-Harris 1994).

These discs are made up of a central, gelatinous nucleus pulposus that is surrounded by a tough but elastic annulus fibrosis. Collagen fibers continue from the annulus into the adjacent tissues, which ties this structure to each vertebral body at its rim, to the anterior and posterior longitudinal ligaments, and to the cartilaginous endplates superiorly and inferiorly. The nucleus pulposus is a self-contained, pliable gelatinous structure that is approximately 88% water in a healthy young disc. It is essentially a hydraulic system that provides support and separates the vertebrae, absorbs shock, permits transient compression and allows for movement (Roberts *et al.* 2006).

At birth, the intervertebral disc has some vascular supply within both the cartilage endplates and the anulus fibrosus, but these vessels soon recede, leaving the disc with little direct blood supply in the healthy adult (Roberts *et al.* 2006).

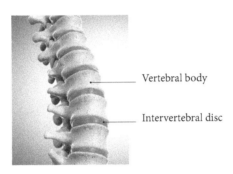

Vertebral body

Intervertebral disc

Intervertebral disc

Deep posterior muscles of the spine

There are many layers of muscles on the posterior aspect of the spine. The deepest layer of muscles attaches only to the vertebrae: the intertransverse muscles connect adjacent transverse processes along the lumbar spine; the interspinales muscles connect adjacent spinous processes along the length of the spine; and the transversospinalis muscles originate at the transverse processes of the vertebrae and lie along the entire length of the spine. The transversospinalis muscles are made up of three different groups of muscles: the rotatores which lie mainly in the thoracic region and pass towards the spinous process of the vertebra above; the multifidus which insert on the spinous process two vertebrae above; and the semispinalis muscles which insert on the spinous process of the vertebra four to six levels above. While all of these muscles are weakly involved in different spinal movements, they are mainly involved in maintaining stability and alignment of the vertebrae and intervertebral discs. Wilke *et al.* (1995) found that the actions of the multifidi account for more than two-thirds of the stiffness of the spine when in a neutral position.

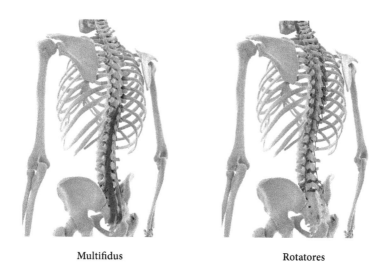

Multifidus   Rotatores

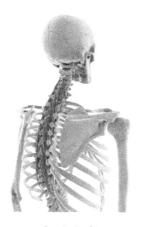

Semispinalis

Intermediate muscles of the back

A collection of muscles known as the erector spinae form a layer superficial to the muscles previously described. They are often referred to as the paraspinal muscles and are made up of three groups: iliocostalis (most lateral); longissimus; and spinalis (most medial). These muscles run more or less the length of the spine. The erector spinae play an important role in maintaining static equilibrium of the trunk by resisting the flexion movement imposed by gravity and any mass carried anterior to the spine. The role of the erector spinae as a tonic muscle group (i.e., fairly resistant to fatigue) has been confirmed by a study by Briggs *et al.* (2004) that found a predominance of type I muscle fibers (slow twitch, associated with endurance) at both thoracic and lumbar levels.

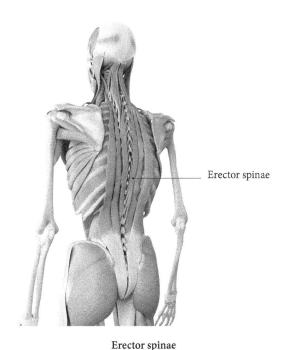

Erector spinae

Erector spinae

Spinal movements

The spine can flex and extend (forward fold and backbend) in the sagittal plane, laterally flex (side bend) in the frontal plane and rotate (twist) in the transverse plane. In the next chapters we will explore the typical range of movement available at each main section of the spine.

LENGTHENING THE SPINE

There is widespread belief that we can lengthen our spine (i.e., actively move the vertebra further apart from each other and grow taller). In fact, there are no muscles that have been shown to be able to draw the vertebrae apart. It is also unclear if traction (e.g., using gravity in a long-held standing forward fold) can increase the space between adjacent vertebrae either.

We do however have the ability to diminish the curves of the spine (i.e., attempt to straighten the spine) and this will have the effect of moving our head further away from our coccyx. It is important to note that it is not possible to completely diminish the curves and therefore fully straighten the spine.

The obsession with the idea of lengthening the spine has probably come about because so many people tend to slouch when they sit or stand. While it doesn't tend to be effective to initiate spinal movements from a slouched position, it often isn't effective to initiate spinal movements from a 'straightened' position either. Moving from a more neutral position might be a better place to start. You can explore your neutral range by slouching followed by straightening and settle with a position in between these two extremes. We will discuss this topic in more detail in Chapter 7 when we will explore the concept of good versus bad posture.

Chapter 6

THE LUMBAR SPINE

The anatomy of the lumbar spine

The lumbar spine is typically comprised of five vertebrae that lie between the pelvis and the ribcage. A study by Hanson *et al.* (2010) reported that 20% of outpatients did not have five lumbar vertebrae: 14.5% had six; 5.3% had four; and one (0.13%) had the rare finding of three lumbar vertebrae.

The lumbar spine supports much of our body weight and the vertebrae are large with thick intervertebral discs to compensate for this. This section of the spine is concave posteriorly because of wedge-shaped intervertebral discs, creating a natural lumbar lordosis. Humans are the only vertebrates to have a lordotic lumbar spine, allowing us to stand on two limbs for prolonged periods.

The lumbar facets are generally oriented in the sagittal plane, favoring the movements of flexion and extension. Kapandji (2010) stated that the shape and the orientation of the superior and inferior facets typically allow for 20° of lateral flexion and 5° of rotation in the lumbar spine. For extension and flexion, the author groups the thoracic and lumbar spine together and states that 60° and 105° are the typical ranges of movement respectively.

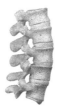

Lumbar vertebrae

The musculature of the lumbar region

Quadratus lumborum (QL) is a deep spinal muscle that originates from the posterior iliac crest and inserts on the lowest rib and the transverse processes of the lumbar vertebrae. It is interesting to note that while various actions on the lumbar spine have been attributed to QL, they have not been substantiated by quantitative data. When the pelvis is fixed, contraction of QL is strongly believed to cause lateral flexion of the lumbar spine and ribcage. Therefore, when the spine and ribs are fixed, contraction is likely to cause the pelvis on that side to rise towards the ribcage. Bilateral contraction of QL may lead to extension of the lumbar spine. QL may also be involved in expiration by acting to pull the ribcage downwards (Gray *et al.* 2005).

While QL is positioned posterolateral to the lumbar spine, psoas major is positioned anterolateral. We have discussed the role of the psoas muscle in hip flexion but the function of the muscle in relation to the spine is an area of controversy and uncertainty in the scientific literature. While some sources describe the psoas as a stabilizer of the lumbar spine, other sources describe its role in flexing the lumbar spine (Penning 2000).

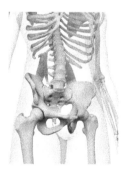

Quadratus lumborum

The abdominal muscles are four paired muscles that fill the area between the ribcage and the pelvis at the front, sides and back. Transversus abdominis (TA) is the deepest of these four muscles. Inferiorly it attaches to the inguinal ligament in the groin and the iliac crest, superiorly to the inner surfaces of the bottom seven ribs and posteriorly to the five lumbar vertebrae. Anteriorly the muscles join to form a flat, broad tendon. This specific tendon that connects muscle to muscle is called an aponeurosis. The fibers of the TA run horizontally around the abdomen. Contraction of the TA decreases the diameter of the abdomen and can be felt during coughing. If the vertebrae are fixed, contraction of the TA pulls the front of the abdomen back towards the spine. If the aponeurosis is fixed, contraction pulls the lumbar spine forward into lordosis. TA is the major contributor for generating expiratory pressure as we exhale (Misuri *et al.* 1997).

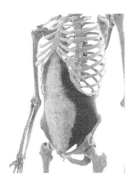

Transversus abdominis

The internal oblique (IO) lies superficial to the TA. Inferiorly it is attached to the inguinal ligament and the iliac crest, superiorly to the lower four ribs. Posteriorly it attaches to the fascia of the deep back muscles and anteriorly it forms a very broad aponeurosis. The fibers of the IO run in an anterosuperior direction (forward and up). Unilateral contraction results in lateral flexion and rotation of the spine and ribcage, drawing the opposite shoulder forwards. When the pelvis is fixed, bilateral contraction causes flexion of the trunk and compression of the abdomen. When the pelvis and the vertebrae are fixed, bilateral contraction pulls the ribs down and posterior. The IO can therefore be recruited during active exhalation.

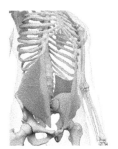

Internal oblique

The external oblique (EO) lies superficial to the IO. Inferiorly it is attached to the ilioinguinal ligament of the pelvis and superiorly to the outer surface of the lower eight ribs. Anteriorly it forms another broad aponeurosis. The fibers run anteroinferior (forward and down, at right angles to those of the IO). Unilateral contraction results in lateral flexion and rotation of the spine and ribcage, drawing the shoulder on that side forward. Bilateral contraction causes flexion of the trunk. When the pelvis is fixed, the lower ribs are pulled down, therefore aiding exhalation. The opposite EO and IO work in synergy with each other.

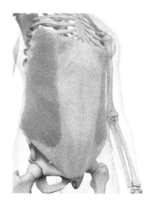

External oblique

The TA, IO and EO not only function to protect the abdominal organs, but also to increase abdominal pressure facilitating defecation, urination and childbirth.

Rectus abdominis is the most superficial of the abdominal muscles and is divided into four parts by a long fibrous band. It runs from the lower sternum and rib cartilage down to the pubic bone. It is involved in flexing the trunk by pulling the sternum towards the pelvis or tilting the pelvis backwards. The common name for the rectus abdominis is the 'six pack' even though there are eight sections of the muscle.

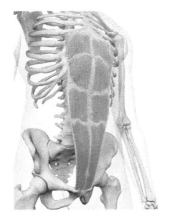

Rectus abdominis

WHAT IS MEANT BY THE 'CORE'?

It is worth noting that there are many different definitions of the 'core' musculature depending on the source and context. Sometimes the core is simply thought of as the four layers of abdominal muscles that we have just explored. We can think about the core in more detail as the musculature that surrounds the lumbopelvic region. This would include the abdominal muscles anteriorly, the deep muscles of the spine and gluteal muscles posteriorly, the pelvic-floor musculature inferiorly, the hip abductors and rotators laterally, and the diaphragm superiorly.

Common lumbar spine injuries and conditions

In this section we will explore some of the most common lumbar spine injuries and conditions that affect our population.

Nonspecific lower back pain (LBP)

Nonspecific LBP can be defined as LBP not attributed to recognizable, known, specific pathology. LBP is the second most common cause of disability in US adults (Centers for Disease Control and Prevention (CDC)

2001). Over 80% of the population will experience an episode of LBP at some time during their life (Rubin 2007). Peak prevalence is believed to occur between 35 and 55 years of age (Andersson 1997).

According to Kinkade (2007) the source of acute LBP cannot be identified in 80% of patients. Approximately 4% of people seen with LBP in primary care have compression fractures and fewer than 1% have a tumor. Ankylosing spondylitis and spinal infections are even rarer. Herniated discs account for only 4% of LBP cases.

Although several potential risk factors have been identified, the causes of the onset of LBP remain obscure and diagnosis difficult to make. A systematic literature review by Bakker *et al.* (2009) found strong evidence that leisure time sport or exercises, sitting, and prolonged standing and/or walking are not associated with LBP. They stated that evidence for associations in leisure time activities (e.g., home repair, gardening), nursing tasks, heavy physical work and working with one's trunk in a bent and/or twisted position and LBP was conflicting. Psychosocial risk factors may include stress, distress, anxiety, depression, cognitive dysfunction, pain behavior, job dissatisfaction and mental stress at work (van Tulder *et al.* 2006).

The association between severe spinal degeneration found using diagnostic imaging and nonspecific LBP is weak. Van Tulder *et al.* (2006) suggested that diagnostic imaging tests should not be used if there are no clear indications of possible serious pathology or radicular syndrome (pain and other symptoms such as numbness, tingling and weakness in the arms or legs).

Acute LBP is usually self-limiting (90% recovery rate within six weeks) but 2–7% of people are thought to develop persistent pain (van Tulder *et al.* 2006).

Osteoarthritis (OA) of the spine and degenerative disc disease

OA of the spine involves the facet joints of the vertebrae and is intimately linked to the distinct but functionally related condition of degenerative disc disease, which affects structures in the anterior aspect of the vertebral column. It is often referred to as spondylosis.

Intervertebral discs degenerate far earlier than other musculoskeletal tissues do; the first unequivocal findings of degeneration in the lumbar discs have been found in the age group 11–16 years. A systematic literature review by Brinjikji *et al.* (2015) found that the prevalence of disc degeneration in asymptomatic individuals increased from 37% of 20-year-old individuals to 96% of 80-year-old individuals. In comparison, they found facet degeneration in 4% of 20-year-old individuals, but the prevalence again increased sharply with age to 83% of 80-year-old individuals.

Annular fissures, which are separations between the annular fibers or separations of annular fibers from their attachments to the vertebral bone, are a feature of disc degeneration. Sometimes these are referred to as 'annular tears', which has the inappropriate connotation of injury as a cause.

Major changes in disc behavior have a strong influence on other spinal structures and may affect their function and predispose them to injury. For instance, as a result of the rapid loss of disc height under load in degenerate discs, the adjacent facet joints may be subject to abnormal loads and eventually develop osteoarthritic changes.

It is important to note that there is no consensus in the scientific literature as to the exact definition of 'disc degeneration' or how it should be distinguished from the physiologic processes of growth, aging, healing and adaptive remodeling. Many health professionals prefer to use the term 'age-related' instead of 'degenerative' due to the negative connotations connected to this word.

As mentioned previously, the association between severe spinal degeneration found using diagnostic imaging and nonspecific LBP is weak (van Tulder *et al.* 2006).

Intervertebral disc pathologies

An intervertebral disc herniation occurs when part of a disc pushes outward beyond its normal boundaries. Medical professionals use several terms to describe the extent or phase of a disc herniation seen on an MRI examination: disc protrusion, disc extrusion and disc sequestration. This classification depends on the condition of the annulus fibrosus and the nucleus pulposus.

A paper by Fardon *et al.* (2014) provides a resource that promotes a clear understanding of lumbar disc terminology among clinicians, radiologists and researchers: in a disc protrusion the disc and associated ligaments remain intact but form an outpouching that can press against nerves; a disc extrusion occurs when the nucleus squeezes through a weakness or tear in the annulus, but the soft material is still connected to the disc; in a disc sequestration the nucleus not only squeezes out but also separates from the main part of the disc. This is also known as a 'free fragment'. Both a disc extrusion and sequestration can trigger an immune response and inflammation.

While the terms 'bulging' and 'herniated' are often used interchangeably, there are clinical distinctions between the two: a herniation measures less than 25% of the total disc circumference while a bulge measures more than 25% of the total disc circumference.

The vast majority of bulges or herniations occur in the posterior direction and slightly laterally (Daghighi *et al.* 2014).

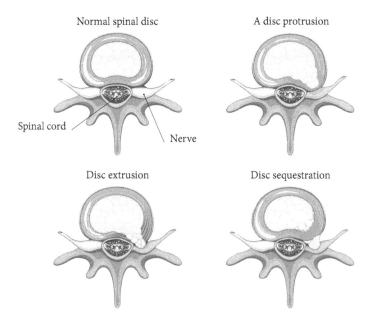

Phases of disc herniation

Our robust intervertebral discs are interwoven with the vertebra and are also supported by many of the spinal ligaments that we have described. The discs themselves cannot 'slip' out of place. A 'ruptured' disc is also not an accepted medical term and suggests trauma when none has occurred. The technical term is 'displacement of disc material'.

As a result of the aging process, increasing amounts of fibrous tissue replace the highly elastic collagen fibers of the younger intervertebral disc. The older disc is less elastic, and its hydraulic recoil mechanism is weakened. The intervertebral disc is avascular by the third decade of life, and nutrition is delivered to the disc by diffusion (Roberts *et al.* 2006).

It has been suggested that the narrowing of the posterior longitudinal ligament in the lumbar spine inadequately reinforces the lumbar discs, which creates an inherent structural weakness (Devereaux 2009). This narrowing, coupled with the great static and kinetic stress placed on the lumbar discs, may contribute to their susceptibility to herniation. Ohshima *et al.* (1993) suggested that the phase of disc herniation is related to variation of the posterior longitudinal ligament. Dixit (2017) proposed that the lumbosacral spine is susceptible to disc herniation because of its mobility. The author stated that 75% of flexion and extension in this region occurs at the lumbosacral joint (L5–S1) and 20% occurs at L4–5, and 90–95% of clinically significant compressive radiculopathies (irritation to nerve roots) occur at these two levels.

Deyo (2002) and Jarvik *et al.* (2005) stated that disc bulges and herniations are highly prevalent in pain-free populations, are not strongly predictive of future LBP and correlate poorly with levels of pain and disability. One literature review showed that in a group of 20-year-olds who were not experiencing back pain, 30% had bulging intervertebral discs (Brinjikji *et al.* 2015). A second review reported that in a group of 50-year-olds who were not experiencing back pain, 60% had bulging discs (Beattie 2008).

It is suggested that herniated discs account for only 4% of LBP cases (Kinkade 2007). There is debate in the literature regarding nociceptive nerve supply to the intervertebral disc and what role the disc plays as a generator of back pain. Studies by Korkala *et al.* (1985) and Palmgren *et al.* (1999) lend support to the concept that the normal intervertebral disc is almost without nerve innervation.

A systematic review of the literature by Chiu *et al.* (2015) found that 50% of patients had spontaneous resolution of herniated discs after conservative treatment. They also report that patients with disc extrusion and sequestration had a significantly higher possibility of having spontaneous regression than did those with bulging or protruding discs. Disc sequestration had a significantly higher rate of complete regression than did disc extrusion. Therefore, the more severe the herniation the greater the chance of spontaneous resolution.

Osteoporosis

Osteoporosis is a systemic skeletal condition characterized by low bone mass and microarchitectural deterioration of bone tissue that increases bone fragility and risk for fractures (US Department of Health and Human Services (DoHHS) 2004).

Osteoporosis may occur without a known cause, or secondary to another condition including corticosteroid therapy, excessive alcohol use, low calcium intake, vitamin D deficiency, smoking, antiepileptic drug use, thyrotoxicosis, primary hyperparathyroidism, chronic liver or kidney disease, rheumatoid arthritis and diabetes.

Osteoporosis is diagnosed in individuals on the basis of the presence of a fragility fracture or by bone mass measurement criteria. A fragility fracture results from forces that would not normally cause a fracture, such as a hip or wrist fracture from falling from standing height or a vertebral compression fracture. Although specific fracture sites have been considered more characteristic of osteoporosis, fractures occurring at nearly every anatomical site have been associated with osteoporosis. It is estimated that 30–50% of women and 15–30% of men will have an osteoporotic fracture in their lifetime (US DoHHS 2004).

Lumbar hyperlordosis

Polly *et al.* (1996) suggested that normal lumbar lordosis is characterized by an average lumbosacral angle of between 39° and 53°. Been and Kalichman (2014) stated that there is evidence that many factors such as age, gender, body mass index, ethnicity and physical activity may affect the lordosis angle, making it difficult to determine uniform normal values. When the curvature of the lumbar spine is very pronounced it is referred to as hyperlordotic.

Norton, Sahrmann and Van Dillen (2004) found that the lumbar lordosis angle was 13.2° larger for women than for men. They found no difference in lumbar curvature between people with and without LBP. Been and Kalichman (2014) suggested that there is evidence that the lumbar lordosis angle is positively and significantly associated with spondylolysis and spondylolisthesis (we will discuss these conditions next). However, they report that inconclusive evidence exists for association between lordosis and LBP, and no association was found with other spinal degenerative features.

Spondylolysis

Spondylolysis (not to be confused with spondylosis, which is a synonym for OA) is defined as unilateral or bilateral fracture of the vertebral facet joints. This occurs almost exclusively in the lower lumbar region, most often at L5 (Fredrickson *et al.* 1984). A small study by Kalichman *et al.* (2009) reported that the prevalence of lumbar spondylolysis in an unselected adult community-based population was 11.5%. The male-to-female ratio was approximately 3:1 and no significant association was identified between spondylolysis (or spondylolisthesis) and the occurrence of LBP.

The exact cause of spondylolysis remains unclear. The most accepted theory is repetitive mechanical stress, specifically lumbar extension and rotation, which results in overuse or stress fracture (Berger and Doyle 2019).

Spondylolisthesis

Spondylolisthesis is the displacement of one vertebra relative to another in the sagittal plane and can be graded based upon the degree of the displacement. Isthmic spondylolisthesis is associated with spondylolysis while degenerative spondylolisthesis is associated with degeneration of the facet joints and/or intervertebral discs. Isthmic spondylolisthesis occurs most often at the L5–S1 junction (Wiltse and Winter 1983) while degenerative spondylolisthesis occurs most often at the L4–5 junction (Fitzgerald and Newman 1976).

Kalichman *et al.* (2009) found that the male-to-female ratio was 2:1 for isthmic spondylolisthesis and 1:3 for degenerative spondylolisthesis. They state that the prevalence of degenerative spondylolisthesis showed a statistically significant increase with age, as can be expected. The relationship between spondylolisthesis and clinically significant LBP has been the subject of ongoing controversy.

Lumbar spinal stenosis

Lumbar spinal stenosis is characterized by narrowing of the spinal canal, which may occur in the central spinal canal, in the area under the facet joints or more laterally, in the intervertebral foramina. Acquired degenerative stenosis is the most frequently observed type of spinal stenosis. It arises in conjunction with age-associated degeneration of the lumbar discs and facet joints. The degenerative process leads to a loss of disc height with associated bulging of the disc and in-folding of the ligamentum flavum. Stenosis may also arise in the setting of spondylolisthesis.

Compression of nerve roots causes symptomatic lumbar spinal stenosis, although the underlying mechanism is not fully understood. Evidence suggests that in the presence of stenosis and nerve root compression, lumbar extension reduces the cross-sectional area of the central canal as well as the intervertebral foramina, exerting further pressure on the blood vessels surrounding the nerve roots. This process may then lead to ischemic (reduction of blood flow) nerve impairment. This ischemic mechanism may account for the typical reversibility of symptoms when patients flex their spines forward (Katz and Harris 2008).

Although the incidence and prevalence of symptomatic lumbar spinal stenosis have not been established, this condition is the most frequent indication for spinal surgery in patients older than 65 years of age (Ciol *et al.* 1996).

Diastasis of rectus abdominis muscle (DRAM)

DRAM is a condition that occurs during and after pregnancy in which the two rectus muscles are separated by an abnormal distance due to stretching and thinning of the linea alba (the fibrous structure that runs down the midline of the abdomen). An increase in the inter-recti distance can weaken the abdominal muscles (Liaw *et al.* 2011) and disturb their functions in lumbopelvic stability (Khushboo, Amrit and Mahesh 2014). A couple of small studies have reported an association with DRAM and pelvic-floor dysfunction and LBP (Spitznagle, Leon and Dillen 2007 and Khushboo *et al.* 2014 respectively).

Varying estimates of the incidence of DRAM have been reported ranging from 66% to 100% during the third trimester of pregnancy (Benjamin, van de Water and Peiris 2014). Despite DRAM being a common and significant clinical problem, little is known about its prevention or management.

IS SPINAL FLEXION BAD?

Yoga sequences often feature a lot of 'chest/heart openers' and twists but do not tend to feature so much active flexion of the spine. A common justification for not focusing so much on spinal flexion in yoga classes can be that since so many us tend to sit in a position of passive flexion for most of the day, at our desks or in our cars, our focus should be on backbends to balance this out. This also goes along with theory that to 'correct' a slouched sitting posture we must simply stretch the front of the abdomen and chest and strengthen the back body.

In reality things just aren't that simple. We need to keep moving our spine in its *full* range of motion in a controlled way to keep it healthy. This includes active flexing, extending, side bending and twisting. If we avoid flexing altogether our spines can become 'flexion intolerant' (meaning that we begin to lose the ability to flex). And in terms of our musculature and soft tissue it is often more effective to stretch *and* strengthen the front, the back and the sides of the abdomen and chest.

There is also the widespread belief that flexion is simply bad for our spines and that this movement is the culprit in terms of 'slipped' discs and LBP. Common phrases in everyday life such as

'Watch your back' or 'I've got your back' can add to the incorrect idea that our spines are inherently fragile. This set of fear-based beliefs sets people up with negative expectations, which has been linked to poorer outcomes and greater pain (Bialosky, Bishop and Cleland 2010). Evidence suggests that fear-avoidance beliefs are prognostic for poor outcome in patients with LBP and should be addressed in this population to avoid delayed recovery (Wertli *et al.* 2014). A systematic review by Saraceni *et al.* (2019) reported that there is (low-quality) evidence that greater lumbar spine flexion during lifting is not a risk factor for LBP onset/persistence, nor a differentiator of people with and without LBP.

The reality is that spinal flexion is a natural movement that is involved in so many of our everyday activities and it really can't be avoided. I'm not suggesting that we all suddenly start picking up really heavy objects with fully flexed spines, but if we only ever lift a load with a more neutral spine then we only become efficient at making that particular movement pattern.

While spinal flexion for one student who has a prolapsed disc might not feel so good, it can often feel perfectly fine for another person with the same condition. An individualized approach is key.

It is worth noting that while people who have osteoporosis will benefit from gentle spinal movement, there needs to be a degree of caution here, due to the increased risk of vertebral fracture. Spinal flexion, extension, rotation and lateral flexion should all be practiced in a particularly mindful, gentle and controlled way while limiting the range of movement. Rolling up from a standing forward fold can put a significant amount of stress on each level of the spine during the transition, so a good option here is to place the hands at the back of the legs to reduce the load or to rise up with a more neutral spine and the hands on the hips.

In the previous chapter we discussed the fact that we are tallest first thing in the morning when the intervertebral discs are their most plump, and we slowly become shorter during the day as the discs subtly flatten under our body weight (Botsford *et al.* 1994). Snook *et al.* (1998) suggested that limiting spinal flexion early in the morning is a form of self-care for people with persistent, nonspecific LBP and can potentially reduce pain. A study by Fathallah, Marras and Wright (1995) reported similar results and concluded that risk of injury was also greater early in the day when disc hydration was at a high level.

Nothing is ever black and white when it comes to movement. The key is to keep exploring all of the movement options that we have available to us, listening to our bodies and making changes when a movement doesn't work so well for us or give us the desired outcome.

Key yoga asanas and how to adapt them

We will now explore some asanas that may present a challenge to students who are affected by the common injuries or conditions that we have discussed above and look at some of the ways that these can be adapted in order to make them more accessible.

Backbends

In Camel Pose (Ustrasana) hug a blanket or foam block between your thighs and either keep your hands on your hips or place your hands on your lower back as you extend. Placing a bolster on top of the ankles can add welcome support for those of you who want to reach your arms back. Remember that this asana can also be practiced from a chair.

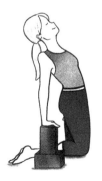

Camel Pose

Cobra Pose (Bhujangasana) or Sphinx Pose (Salamba Bhujangasana) are good alternatives to Upward Facing Dog (Urdhva Mukha Svanasana). In Cobra Pose the pelvis remains in contact with the floor and in Sphinx Pose the forearms support the upper body. A great option is to practice these asanas standing against a wall.

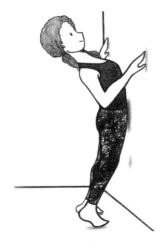

Cobra Pose

In Bridge Pose (Setu Bandha Sarvangasana) gently hug a blanket or foam block between your thighs and use the support of a bolster or stack of foam blocks underneath your pelvis.

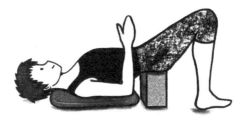

Bridge Pose

SHOULD WE ENGAGE THE GLUTEAL MUSCLES DURING A BACKBEND?

'Relax your glutes' has become a common cue for many teachers when teaching backbends. It is difficult to ascertain exactly where this cue originated from and why. Backbends typically involve the whole body, with activation of the entire posterior chain of muscles. The majority of backbends involve hip extension which is one of the main roles of the gluteus maximus. The hamstrings also extend the hip, but if the knees are bent (like in backbends such as Wheel Pose, Urdhva Dhanurasana) then they are already in a shortened position and won't play such a big role in hip extension. So, in reality it is impossible to backbend without the use of gluteus maximus.

Engaging the gluteus maximus also moves the focal point of the backbend away from the lumbar spine and to the pelvis, which is a more stable structure. This also prevents us from simply taking the path of least resistance, i.e., making most of the movement come from the lumbar spine and not making the most of hip extension and thoracic extension. The more we use the gluteus maximus the stronger it becomes, which is great for those of us who have weakness here.

It is important to note that a balanced action is helpful here, otherwise we can potentially create too much tension at the back of the pelvis. This can be achieved by initiating some internal rotation of the hips to counterbalance the external rotation that is also initiated by the gluteus maximus. In Bridge Pose we could create some internal rotation in the hip joints before we lift the pelvis by energetically drawing the feet apart (without actually moving them). It is also helpful to recognize if we are clenching or gripping the gluteus maximus instead of simply engaging it. The breath is often the clue here, so notice if you are holding your breath or unable to breathe fully. When we clench the gluteus maximus, we often clench our jaw too.

Forward folds

In Standing Forward Fold (Uttanasana) or Wide Leg Forward Fold (Prasarita Padottanasana) bend your knees gently and either rest your hands on your thighs or on a chair or set of stacked foam blocks in front of you.

In Seated Forward Fold (Paschimottanasana) rest a rolled-up blanket underneath your knees and raise your seat by sitting on a blanket or cushion. Instead of reaching your arms up, which will add to the load on your lumbar spine, walk your hands forward as you fold.

In Bound Angle Pose (Baddha Konasana) and Wide-Angle Seated Forward Bend (Upavistha Konasana) raising your seat with a foam block, cushion or folded blanket is a good start.

A rolled-up blanket under the outer thighs can be a great support in Bound Angle Pose, particularly for the restorative version of the asana. Move slowly and mindfully. In Wide-Angle Seated Forward Bend you can rest your arms and forehead on a chair or stack of foam blocks in front of you.

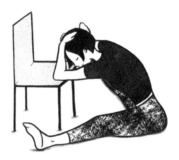

Wide-Angle Seated Forward Bend

Twists

At the start of the chapter we discussed that there is approximately 5° of rotation available in the lumbar spine. In asanas that involve rotation of the spine, it is important to remember that the majority of this movement will be coming from the thoracic and cervical spine, and not the lumbar spine. It can be helpful to imagine the spine as a spiral staircase growing larger with each step.

In supine twists it can feel more supportive to stabilize the pelvis and move the upper body instead of stabilizing the upper body and moving the pelvis. Start by lying on your side with your hip bones stacked. You can gently squeeze a blanket between your thighs and begin to roll your top shoulder back towards the floor. If your shoulder and arm do not comfortably rest on the floor they can be supported with a blanket, cushion or bolster. Another option is to straighten your bottom leg in line with your spine and rest your top knee and shin onto a bolster.

In twists it is helpful to focus on mobility over flexibility (we will discuss this principle in more detail in Chapter 10). It can be easy to rely on external force to move us into twists and to hold us in position, but we therefore miss the opportunity to use our core musculature to do the work and risk applying too much force to our lumbar spine. In seated twists, and in standing twists such as Revolved Chair (Parivrtta Utkatasana), slowly rotate your spine and upper body without using your opposite arm as a lever. Once you are in position you can rest your opposite arm against your leg to help maintain length in your spine but ideally you should be able to stay in position if you release your arm.

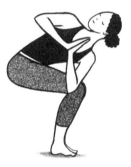

Revolved Chair

Side bends

At the start of the chapter we discussed that there is approximately 20° of lateral flexion available in the lumbar spine. In the next chapter we will discuss how there is a similar range of lateral flexion in the thoracic spine. In asanas that involve lateral flexion of the spine, it is important to utilize the full length of the spine rather than simply hinging at the waist. Attempting to keep length in both sides of the waist can be helpful here.

Improving the overall health of the lumbar spine

This section addresses some effective ways in which we can all improve and maintain the health and functioning of our lumbar spine. It is intended to be a general guide for yoga practitioners and teachers and is not a replacement for the personal advice of a health professional.

Movement is medicine

A detailed report aimed at primary care physicians by van Tulder *et al.* (2006) suggested that an active approach is the best treatment option for acute LBP. The group recommended that the advice to stay active or to get active should be promoted, and that an increase in fitness will improve general health. A systematic review by McCaffrey and Park (2012) looked at the benefits of yoga for musculoskeletal disorders including osteoporosis. Noting that they were only able to include three studies on osteoporosis in their review due to their inclusion criteria, they reported that yoga has a positive impact on osteoporosis. A ten-year study by Lu *et al.* (2016) suggested that yoga can reverse bone loss that has reached the stages of osteoporosis. A systematic review by Sharma and Haider (2013a) found that a reduction in LBP can be achieved by using yoga as part of the intervention. A systematic review by Cramer *et al.* (2013a) found strong evidence for short-term effectiveness and moderate evidence for long-term effectiveness of yoga for chronic LBP. A systematic review by Wieland *et al.* (2017) concluded that there is low- to moderate-certainty evidence that yoga compared to non-exercise controls results in small to moderate improvements in back-related function at three and six months.

Our bodies have evolved to move. As I mentioned in the earlier discussion on spinal flexion, we need to keep moving our spine in its full range of (pain-free) motion, in a controlled way, to keep it healthy. This includes active flexing, extending, side bending and twisting. So, whether it is yoga, Pilates, Zumba, pole dancing or just jumping around your room in your underwear, keep it up! In the next chapter we will explore the social concept of 'good posture'. It is my strong belief that it is not how we sit or stand that impacts the health of our spine but the fact that if we are sitting or standing for prolonged periods then we are not moving our spines.

If you drive a lot or sit at a desk for hours every day, take regular short breaks to move and stretch. Seated Cat-Cow Pose (Chakravakasana) is a really accessible pose that can be practiced pretty much anywhere.

1. Sit on a chair with your feet roughly hip-distance wide and under your knees.

2. Slowly rock your pelvis back and forward.

3. Then begin to make circular movements with your pelvis in both directions.

4. Interlace your fingers behind your head or place your hands on your shoulders and slowly side bend in each direction.

5. Try to focus more on how controlled you can make the full range of movement rather than aiming to get straight into a position of stretch.

Isolating lumbar spine movements

In my own personal experience and from my experience of teaching movement for over a decade, I can testify that focusing on specific, precise spinal movements can work wonders for the health of the spine.

The Cat-Cow Pose options that we discussed in Chapter 4 work equally well here since the areas are so intimately connected.

1. Lie on your back with your knees bent and feet flat.

2. Very slowly begin to tilt your pelvis back and forward. This can be thought of as Supine Cat-Cow Pose.

3. Start to become aware of how you are controlling these movements.

4. The mat and floor will help to provide feedback so that you can become more aware of the positions of your pelvis and lumbar spine.

5. Now begin to roll your pelvis clockwise, tilting it forward, to the right, backwards and to the left.

6. Initiate the movements by pressing your feet down and then see if you can roll your pelvis without pressing through your feet.

7. After a few repetitions, repeat this in the opposite direction.

Let's now explore some further Cat-Cow Pose variations.

1. Start on your hands and knees.

2. Move as slowly as you can through the gentle flexion and extension sequence.

3. Start to become more aware of how you are actually making these subtle movements happen. Begin to make pelvic circles in one direction and then the opposite direction, controlling each subtle movement.

4. Stay within pain-free range.

5. Come back to a neutral position on your hands and knees.

6. Try to stabilize your upper spine and attempt to only move your lower spine and pelvis as you practice Cat-Cow Pose again. This can take time and patience.

7. Rest for a moment.

8. Now begin to draw your right hip bone up to meet your lower ribs.

9. At the same time draw your ribcage down to meet your right hip bone.

10. Slowly move back to a neutral position and repeat this on the other side.

11. Repeat this sequence slowly a few times, breathing smoothly.

12. Notice the differences between the right and left side.

Core stability

'Working the core' has become a huge focus of rehabilitation of athletes and nonathletes in recent years. The belief that the spine's stabilizing muscles become inhibited with back pain, rendering the spine unstable and vulnerable, often drives this. It is worth noting that growing evidence tells us that persistent back pain disorders are often associated with increased trunk muscle co-contraction, earlier activation of the transverse abdominal wall and an inability to relax the stabilizing muscles of the spine such as lumbar multifidus (Dankaerts *et al.* 2009; Geisser *et al.* 2004; Gubler *et al.* 2010). So, while we will look at a couple of common 'core stability' exercises, it is worth noting that focusing on periods of relaxation for these muscles is also important. Restorative yoga practices are a great option here. Recent studies have also demonstrated that positive outcomes associated with stabilization training are best predicted by reductions in catastrophizing[1] rather than changes in muscle patterning (Mannion *et al.* 2012), highlighting that nonspecific factors such as therapeutic alliance and confidence in the physical therapist may be the active ingredient in the treatment, rather than the desired change in muscle.

EXERCISE ONE

1. Come onto your hands and knees with a neutral spine.

2. Brace your abdomen and slowly lift your knees a couple of inches off the mat.

3. Keep your pelvis and lumbar spine stabilized.

4. Hold this position for a couple of breaths.

5. Slowly lower your knees back to the floor.

6. Repeat this a couple of times, eventually increasing the length of the hold.

---

1   Catastrophizing is a cognitive process whereby a person exhibits an exaggerated notion of negativity, assuming the worst outcomes and interpreting even minor problems as major calamities (Biggs, Meulders and Vlaeyen 2016).

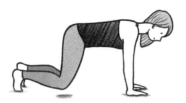

Tabletop Pose with knee hover

EXERCISE TWO

1. Lie on your side with your elbow under your shoulder and your forearm flat on the floor and perpendicular to your body.

2. Stack your hip bones and keep your hips and ankles roughly in the same line as your spine.

3. You have the option to keep your legs straight or bend your knees slightly.

4. Press actively down into your forearm so that you lift up out of your shoulder joint slightly.

5. Brace your abdomen and slowly lift your pelvis up off the mat.

6. Hold this position for a few breaths and then slowly lower.

7. Repeat this a few times or begin to lift and lower repeatedly without holding the position at the top.

8. Repeat this exercise on the other side.

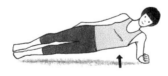

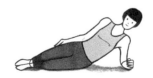

Side Plank variations

Sitting on an exercise ball is another effective way to develop core strength and stability. You can even work up to slowly lifting one foot off the floor at a time and eventually closing your eyes to challenge your balance.

Chapter 7

THE THORACIC SPINE

The anatomy of the thoracic spine

The thoracic spine lies in the region of the thorax or chest, which is designed to protect many important organs including the heart and lungs. The joints and muscles in this region must also be sufficiently mobile and coordinated to function as a mechanical chamber for breathing, which includes coughing and forced exhalation.

The thoracic vertebrae

There are typically 12 thoracic vertebrae; however, just as we have discussed with the coccyx, the sacrum and the lumbar spine, there can be variation here. According to Glass *et al.* (2002) approximately 5–8% of individuals lack a pair of ribs and subsequent thoracic vertebrae. In a study by Yan *et al.* (2018) 6% of the cohort had 11 thoracic vertebrae.

The thoracic vertebrae have thin discs compared to the lumbar region and longer spinous processes. The thoracic facets are generally oriented in the frontal plane. Kapandji (2010) stated that the shape and the orientation of the superior and inferior facets typically allow for 20° of lateral flexion and 35° of rotation in the thoracic spine. For extension and flexion, the author groups the thoracic and lumbar spine together and states that 60° and 105° are the typical ranges of movement respectively. It is important to note that there is no consensus among researchers regarding the typical range of movement at various levels of the vertebral column, but the figures can serve to show that each section is designed to move differently.

Masharawi *et al.* (2004) stated that asymmetry in facet orientation is a normal characteristic in the thoracic spine and report that right thoracic facets are more vertically and frontally oriented than the left ones. They suggested that flexion or extension in the thoracic facets will be coupled with right lateral flexion, ending with a rotational movement.

The thoracic vertebrae are also distinguished by the presence of additional facets on the sides of the vertebral bodies for articulation with the heads of the ribs, and facets on the transverse processes of all except the 11th and 12th vertebrae for articulation with the tubercles of the ribs. These additional facets are often called demifacets. The demifacets are bilaterally paired and located on the superior and inferior posterolateral aspects of the vertebrae. They are positioned so that the superior demifacet of inferior vertebrae articulates with the head of the same rib that articulates with the inferior demifacet of a superior rib. For example, the inferior demifacets of T4 and the superior demifacets of T5 articulate with the head of the fifth rib.

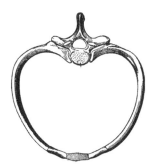

Pair of ribs articulating with the sternum and a thoracic vertebra

The ribcage

The ribcage typically consists of 12 pairs of ribs, 12 vertebrae and the sternum (breastbone). The ribs are labeled one to twelve, with one being the most superior. It was traditionally assumed from the Biblical story of Adam and Eve that men's ribs would number one fewer than women's, until this was controversially proved incorrect by anatomists in the 16th century.

The superior seven ribs are called the 'true ribs' because they articulate with T1 to T7 posteriorly and articulate directly with the sternum anteriorly. The next three ribs are called the 'false ribs' because while they articulate with T8 to T10 posteriorly, they only attach to the cartilage of the seventh rib anteriorly. The inferior two ribs are called the 'floating ribs' because while they articulate with T11 to T12 posteriorly, they have no anterior attachment.

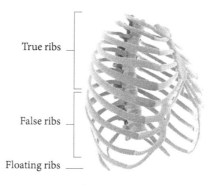

True ribs

False ribs

Floating ribs

The ribcage

The head of each rib has one or two facets for articulation with the demi-facets on the bodies of thoracic vertebrae. The first, tenth, eleventh and twelfth ribs have a single facet on their head that only articulates with its respective vertebra. The second rib through to the ninth rib all have two facets on their heads; the superior facet articulates with the vertebra above the rib, while the inferior facet articulates with the respectively named vertebra. In addition, the first rib through to the tenth rib have tubercles with facets that articulate with the costal (meaning 'rib') facet of the transverse process of each respective vertebra. The eleventh and twelfth ribs have no tubercle and therefore do not articulate with the transverse process of their respective vertebra (Donley and Loyd 2019).

Elevation of the ribs increases the diameter of the chest cavity during inhalation while the lowering of the ribs decreases the diameter during exhalation. The eleventh and twelfth ribs move like calipers to create more space in the lower thorax (Kapandji 2010).

The sternum is a vertical bone that forms the anterior and central portion of the chest wall. The sternum is divided anatomically into three sections: the manubrium, the body and the xiphoid process. The manubrium is the widest section and contains the clavicular notches which articulate with the two clavicles (collar bones). The sternal angle is where the manubrium joins the body of the sternum. The second rib attaches at this point. The xiphoid process is attached inferiorly to the body of the sternum and provides an attachment point for the diaphragm and rectus abdominis, but no ribs.

The muscles of the thorax

The diaphragm is a large, flat, dome-like muscle that inserts on its own central tendon (aponeurosis) and separates the thorax and the abdomen. It originates from the inner sternum and xiphoid process, the inner surface of the lower six ribs and the superior lumbar spine. The diaphragm has fascial connections to the transverse abdominis, quadratus lumborum and psoas muscles.

There are three main openings (hiatuses) in the diaphragm that allow important structures to pass between the thorax and the abdomen. The inferior vena cava (IVC) hiatus contains the IVC and branches of the right phrenic nerve. It passes through the midportion of the central tendon. This opening enlarges with inspiration, drawing blood into the heart. The esophageal hiatus contains the esophagus, vagus nerve and sympathetic nerve branches. It functions as a sphincter by constricting with inspiration and therefore helping to prevent gastroesophageal reflux. The aortic hiatus contains the aorta and the lymphatic thoracic duct. Diaphragmatic contractions do not affect this hiatus.

The diaphragm is the primary muscle of inspiration. Contraction expands the volume of the thoracic cavity, decreasing intrathoracic pressure and drawing air into the lungs. With relaxation of the diaphragm, the elastic recoil of the lungs predominates, causing exhalation. In addition, the diaphragm aids in urination and defecation by increasing intra-abdominal pressure.

During normal respiration a symmetrical change in the pelvic floor can be observed (Talasz *et al.* 2011). During inspiration as the diaphragm subtly descends there is a corresponding lowering of the pelvic floor. This process is thought to have the aim of controlling (and responding to) any change in intra-abdominal pressure. It also ensures the steadiness of the human trunk and maintains urinary continence during respiration and coughing. Talasz *et al.* (2011) stated that before inhalation, electrical activity can be observed in the muscles of the pelvic floor, and the same electrical activity is traceable for the transverse abdominis and internal oblique muscles.

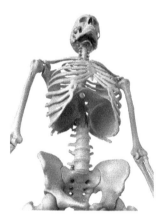

The diaphragm

The intercostal muscles are arranged in three layers between adjacent ribs, with their fibers running perpendicular to the ribs. They consist of the external intercostal, internal intercostal and innermost intercostal muscles. The external intercostal muscles are involved in inhalation while the internal intercostal muscles are involved in exhalation. They are known as accessory muscles of respiration.

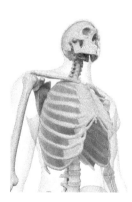

The intercostals

Serratus posterior superior is a thin, four-sided muscle, situated at the superoposterior thorax. It arises from the spinous processes of the seventh cervical and upper two or three thoracic vertebrae and from the supraspinous ligament. Inclining downward and outward, it inserts into the upper borders of the second, third, fourth and fifth ribs.

Serratus posterior inferior is situated at the junction of the thoracic and lumbar regions. It arises from the spinous processes of the lower two thoracic and upper two or three lumbar vertebrae, and from the supraspinous ligament. Passing obliquely upward and outward, it inserts into the inferior borders of the lower four ribs.

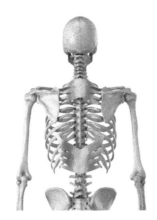

Serratus posterior superior and inferior

The action of these small muscles has been a significant point of controversy amongst anatomists and physiologists alike. While Gray *et al.* (2005) described the role of both muscles in inspiration, Loukas *et al.* (2008) suggested that no respiratory function can be attributed to either the serratus posterior superior or inferior muscles.

INTELLIGENT MOVEMENT PRINCIPLE – GOOD POSTURE IS A SOCIAL CONSTRUCT

There is such widespread belief in the concepts of good and bad posture that we can easily assume that there is an evidence basis for these. To the best of my knowledge there are very few studies that examine the correlation between posture and symptoms. Forward head posture (FHP), commonly known as 'text-neck', is often cited as being one of the leading causes of neck pain but the little research that has been conducted on this topic is inconclusive. In fact, a recent study by Damasceno *et al.* (2018) found no link between HFP and neck pain in a group of 150 young adults.

If you have no choice but to sit or stand all day, then stacking your joints will certainly help you to conserve muscular energy but we also have to recognize that being in one fixed position for prolonged periods is not good for our bodies. I don't believe that it is how we sit that is the problem but the fact that as long as we are sitting, we are not *moving*.

Strong beliefs about the concept of bad posture also reinforce the idea that spinal flexion is inherently problematic. Yoga sequences are filled with 'chest openers' to remedy slouching by simply stretching the front body and strengthening the back body, when most of us would benefit from regularly stretching and strengthening every aspect of the trunk.

I'm not trying to suggest that our posture has no impact on how we feel or that we should suddenly adopt a completely carefree attitude towards it, but it might be time to move away from the idea of an ideal posture and invest our time and energy on moving more.

Common thoracic spine conditions

In this section we will explore some of the most common thoracic spine conditions that affect our population. It is worth noting that since the thoracic spine has less range of movement than the lumbar and cervical spine it is much less prone to injury.

Scoliosis

Scoliosis is a three-dimensional deviation of the spinal axis. The main diagnostic criterion is lateral spinal curvature exceeding 10°.

Scoliosis can be classified as non-idiopathic or idiopathic when an underlying disease has been identified or has not been identified, respectively. The major types of non-idiopathic scoliosis are congenital scoliosis due to malformation or faulty segmentation of the vertebrae and neuromuscular scoliosis due to muscular imbalance.

Scoliosis can also be classified as infantile, juvenile, adolescent or adult depending on the age at which it is first noted. Adult scoliosis can be either a continuation of adolescent idiopathic scoliosis or a recent development owing to degenerative changes or other causes.

A literature review by Trobisch, Suess and Schwab (2010) stated that idiopathic scoliosis is extremely rare in infancy and early childhood but has a prevalence of 1–2% among children up to 15 years of age. Degenerative changes are presumed to account for the further rise in prevalence to over 8% in adults aged 25 and above, and to as high as 68% in persons aged 60–90. Male and female infants are equally affected by infantile scoliosis, but females tend to be more commonly affected with increasing age, so that the sex ratio from age 10 onward is already 6:1. Boys are somewhat more likely than girls to have mild scoliosis, yet the ratio of girls to boys among children with spinal curvatures greater than 20° is 5:1, and it rises to 10:1 in children whose spinal curvature exceeds 30°.

Trobisch *et al.* (2010) also reported that infantile scoliosis frequently corrects itself spontaneously and therefore requires no treatment in over 80% of cases. The remaining cases of progressive scoliosis often require lengthy and complex treatment. They stated that adolescent scoliosis takes a markedly more benign course, and if the angle of deviation does not exceed 20° then the probability of progression is only about 10–20%. The authors found that idiopathic scoliosis rarely causes pain but often comes to attention through a hunched back, lumbar bulging and/or asymmetry of the shoulders, chest and pelvis. However, a study by Jackson, Simmons and Stripinis (1983) found that while adults with scoliosis had a similar incidence of back pain compared to adults without scoliosis, the adults with scoliosis had a greater severity of pain, which increased with age and degree of scoliotic curvature. Bess *et al.* (2009) reported that adults with scoliosis demonstrate greater functional limitations and greater daily analgesic use, and report worse health-related quality of life compared with adults without scoliosis.

It is important to note that the development of scoliosis cannot be prevented. Therefore, attention is currently being focused on early detection, so that timely treatment can be provided to limit progression.

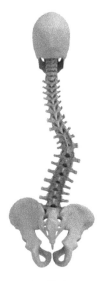

Scoliosis

Thoracic hyperkyphosis

Hyperkyphosis is defined as excessive curvature of the thoracic spine (in the sagittal plane) and may be associated with adverse health effects. Fon, Pitt and Thies (1980) noted that the average thoracic kyphosis increases with age from 20° in childhood, to 25° in adolescents, to 40° in adults.

Ailon *et al.* (2015) suggested that hyperkyphosis has a prevalence of 20–40% and is more common in the geriatric population. They stated that the cause is multifactorial and involves an interaction between degenerative changes, vertebral compression fractures, muscular weakness and altered biomechanics. Schneider *et al.* (2004) reported that although it is commonly assumed that vertebral fractures are responsible for hyperkyphosis, the majority of people with hyperkyphosis do not have vertebral fractures or osteoporosis. They found that degenerative disc disease, not vertebral fractures, was the most common finding associated with hyperkyphosis in men and women.

Greendale *et al.* (2009) stated that adverse health outcomes associated with hyperkyphosis include physical functional limitations, thoracic back pain, respiratory compromise, restricted spinal range of motion and osteoporotic fractures.

IS IT POSSIBLE TO DISLOCATE A RIB?

Although rib subluxations (partial rib dislocations) are claimed to be a common finding by various healthcare professionals, the existence of this condition remains quite controversial.

All of the surrounding connective tissue and musculature are designed to prevent this from happening. To date, there is a lack of radiological evidence supporting the notion that ribs can dislocate and there are no studies that support that a rib subluxation can be reliably diagnosed or treated by manual palpation. There is also no reported evidence that rib subluxations occur even after major traumatic incidences such as a car accident. In a comprehensive review study (Oikonomou and Prassopoulos 2011) on CT scan imaging of patients who had experienced blunt thoracic trauma not one patient was diagnosed with a rib subluxation.

Key yoga asanas and how to adapt them

We will now explore some asanas that may present a challenge to students who are affected by the common conditions that we have discussed above and look at some of the ways that these can be adapted in order to make them more accessible.

Backbends

Cobra Pose (Bhujangasana) or Sphinx Pose (Salamba Bhujangasana) are good alternatives to Upward Facing Dog (Urdhva Mukha Svanasana). In Cobra Pose the pelvis remains in contact with the floor and in Sphinx Pose the forearms support the upper body. A great option is to practice these asanas standing against a wall or seated in a chair.

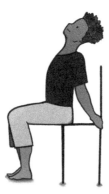

Seated Cobra Pose

Side bends

Seated Crescent Moon is helpful for people who would like more support in their side bend. The seat creates a firm foundation from which one can lift out of and the opposite hand can be used as a support also.

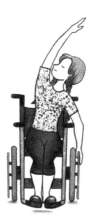

Side bend

In Extended Triangle Pose (Utthita Trikonasana) supporting the lower arm on a chair can help to control the side bend and to maintain more length through both the right and left side body.

Corpse Pose (Savasana)

Savasana is essentially about finding stillness so that we can assimilate our yoga practice. It is important to remember that not everyone feels comfortable lying flat on their back. It can be so easy to have a fixed idea of what Savasana should look like, but really, we can practice Savasana in any comfortable resting position. This can mean being on one's side in the 'fetal position', lying on one's belly or seated with one's back supported by the wall. A supine Savasana can also be supported with blankets and bolsters so that the position becomes truly comfortable and restful.

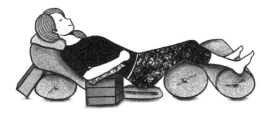

Supported Savasana

Improving the overall health of the thoracic spine

This section addresses some effective ways in which we can work to improve and maintain the health and functioning of our thoracic spine. It is intended to be a general guide for yoga practitioners and teachers and is not a replacement for the personal advice of a health professional.

A randomized controlled trial by Greendale *et al.* (2009) reported significant improvements in hyperkyphosis after a six-month yoga intervention. The active treatment group attended one-hour yoga classes, which consisted of asana and pranayama, three days per week for 24 weeks. The intervention did not result in any statistically significant gains in measured physical performance or in self-assessed health-related quality of life (HRQOL), but the yoga participants reported less upper back pain, early morning awakening and insomnia.

Active and passive twists

We will first explore a gentle twist.

1. In a comfortable seated position cross your arms over your chest.

2. Slowly twist your upper body to the right, keeping your chin in line with your sternum.

3. Twist back to the center and repeat this on the opposite side.

4. Repeat this for a few cycles, moving slowly and mindfully.

5. Adopt whatever breathing pattern feels appropriate for you.

There is now the option to increase the intensity of the twist.

1. Come onto your hands and knees into Tabletop Pose (Bharmanasana).

2. Shift your weight into your left hand.

3. Place your right hand on your right hip, onto your right shoulder or behind your head.

4. Slowly lift up through your right armpit as you start to turn your chest towards the right.

5. Either keep your chin in line with your sternum or slowly turn your head to the right. Control the movement back to the center.

6. Repeat this on the opposite side.

7. Repeat this whole sequence a couple of times.

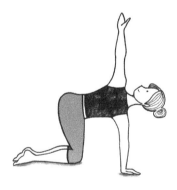

Tabletop twist

There is also the option to make the twist more passive.

1. Back in Tabletop Pose (Bharmanasana) lift up through your right side.

2. Place your right arm under your left waist.

3. Rest your right shoulder and head down onto the mat.

4. If your shoulder or head do not rest comfortably, use the support of a pillow or blanket.

5. After a few breaths in this position slowly support yourself back up onto your hands and knees.

6. Repeat this on the opposite side.

Lateral flexion

We will now explore some simple side bending.

1. Find a comfortable seated position.

2. Either clasp your hands behind your head or place your hands on your shoulders.

3. Slowly lift up out of your waist and up into your armpit as you bend to the right.

4. Control the movement back to center.

5. Repeat this on the opposite side.

6. Repeat this sequence for a few cycles.

7. See how slow and controlled you can make the movements, and, as always, keep your breath smooth and steady.

There is now the option to explore side bending on your hands and knees.

1. Find your Tabletop Pose (Bharmanasana).

2. Begin to draw your right hip bone up to meet your lower ribs.

3. At the same time draw your ribcage down to meet your right hip bone.

4. Slowly move back to a neutral position.

5. Repeat this on the other side.

6. Repeat this sequence slowly a few times.

7. Breathe smoothly and notice the differences between the right and left side.

Cat-Cow isolating thoracic movement

We now explore Cat-Cow focusing on the thoracic spine.

1. Find your comfortable seated position.

2. Slowly begin to lift up through the back of your sternum as you gently backbend.

3. Reverse the movement as you draw your navel back towards your spine and your shoulders forward, rounding your back.

There is the option to use your arms here too.

1. Clasp your hands and turn your palms to face forward.

2. Lift your arms up as you extend your spine.

3. Lower your arms and press your hands forward as you flex your spine.

Let's now explore some further Cat-Cow Pose variations.

1. Come onto your hands and knees.

2. Move as slowly as you can through the gentle flexion and extension sequence.

3. You can also try to initiate the flexion and extension movements by imagining that you are dragging your hands forward and back, respectively.

Become aware of how you are actually making these subtle movements happen and stay within a pain-free range.

1. Come back to a neutral position on your hands and knees.

2. Stabilize your lumbar spine by gently bracing your abdomen.

3. Attempt to only move your thoracic spine as you practice Cat-Cow Pose again.

This can take time and patience. Looping a yoga strap or resistance band across the back of your ribcage is a great way to provide yourself with feedback as you learn to access these specific movements.

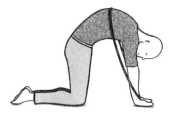

Cat-Cow with resistance band

IS 'FLARING' OF THE RIBS IN A BACKBEND BAD?

Some of us have a natural 'hinge' in our spines, simply meaning that there is a large range of movement available between two particular adjacent vertebrae. It's also possible to have more than one hinge. It can be easy to take the path of least resistance and focus our movements on the areas that already move the most. An example of this would be backbending predominantly at the lumbar–thoracic junction with very little extension throughout the rest of the thoracic spine. This is often called 'flaring' the ribs as the front lower ribs jut forward significantly. This large range of movement at the lumbar–thoracic junction does not necessarily mean that problems will develop in this area, but it is important to ensure that the neighboring vertebrae are moved through their full range too so that each joint remains healthy. Before you begin to extend your spine, gently draw the front of your lower ribs back towards your spine. Then lead the movement by lifting up through your sternum so that the full length of your thoracic spine begins to extend. At this point you can then allow the front of your lower ribs to move forward so that you can access that larger range of movement in the lumbar–thoracic junction.

Improving shoulder girdle mobility

The shoulder girdle and thoracic spine are intimately related and the function of one region will have a great impact on the function of the other. In Chapter 9 we will explore ways to improve the mobility of our shoulder girdles.

Chapter 8

THE CERVICAL SPINE

The anatomy of the cervical spine

The vertebrae of the cervical spine and the base of the cranium interact to provide extensive three-dimensional placement of the head and neck, which is essential for optimal spatial orientation of the special senses (sight, hearing, smell, taste and balance).

The craniovertebral junction (CVJ)

The CVJ is the complex relationship between the occiput (the base of the cranium or skull), C1 and C2. This region houses vital neural and vascular structures while providing the majority of cranial flexion, extension and axial rotation. In fact, the range of movement at the junction exceeds that of any other region of the vertebral column. An intricate combination of bony and ligamentous supports allows for stability despite the large range of movement, while highly specialized muscles control fine movements in the CVJ.

C1 is called the atlas and has no vertebral body or spinous process. It is essentially a bony ring that articulates with the occiput. The predominant movement between the occiput and the atlas is flexion and extension. In fact, it is suggested that this joint makes up about 50% of the flexion and extension range of movement in the cervical region (Bogduk and Mercer 2000).

C2 is called the axis. The axis also lacks a typical vertebral body but has a projecting process called the dens or odontoid process that forms a pivot for the atlas. The predominant movement of the C1–2 vertebral junction is rotation. Again, it is suggested that this joint makes up about 50% of the rotational range of movement in the cervical region (Bogduk and Mercer 2000). There is no intervertebral disc between the atlas and the axis, and this suggests that these vertebrae are not designed to bear weight greater than the head.

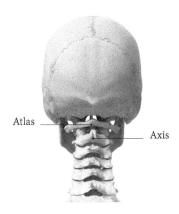

Atlas

Axis

The atlas and the axis

The cervical vertebrae

The cervical spine is made up of seven vertebrae that lie in the region of the neck. Every mammal has seven cervical vertebrae, including the giraffe. The number of cervical vertebrae is very rarely increased or diminished (Gray *et al.* 2005).

C3 to C7 have small vertebral bodies, thick intervertebral discs and short spinous processes. These characteristics contribute to the cervical spine having the greatest range of movement of the entire spine. A significant amount of the range of flexion and extension of the cervical spine occurs at the C5–6 junction. Kapandji (2010) stated that the shape and the orientation of the superior and inferior facets typically allow for 35–40° of lateral flexion, 45–50° of rotation in the cervical spine, 75° of extension and 40° of flexion.

C1 to C6 have a foramen present in each of their transverse processes which encircle the vertebral arteries and veins.

The cervical spine is unique in the fact that different sections can perform different movements simultaneously. A good example of this is Shoulderstand (Salamba Sarvangasana) where the cervical spine is flexed but it is also possible to lift the chin in this position and therefore extend at the CVJ.

Hyoid bone

The hyoid bone forms part of the skeleton of the anterior neck. It does not normally articulate directly with other skeletal structures but is suspended by muscles and ligaments from the occiput and the mandible (lower jawbone) above and connected to the larynx (voice box) and sternum below. It gives attachment to muscles of the tongue, pharyngeal wall and anterior neck from the mandible to the top of the chest. The hyoid bone suspends and anchors the larynx during respiration and speech.

The temporomandibular joint (TMJ)

The TMJ is a complex synovial joint with a capsule and meniscus that connects the mandible with the cranium. The masseter, temporal muscle and the two pterygoids all act on the TMJ.

This joint is connected not only to the cranium but also to the spine and shoulder girdle via soft tissue attachments. It is suggested that cranio-cervical posture is significantly influenced by the TMJ (An *et al.* 2015).

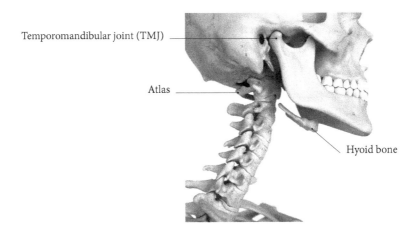

Cervical vertebrae, TMJ and hyoid bone

The musculature of the neck

Sternocleidomastoid (SCM) muscle is present across each side of the neck and forms a prominent landmark when contracted. It originates on the manubrium of the sternum and the clavicle and inserts on the mastoid process behind the ear. Acting alone it laterally flexes the neck and rotates the face to the opposite side. The two muscles acting together flex the head.

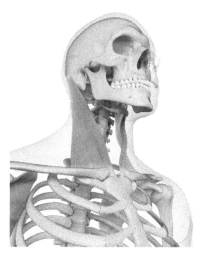

Sternocleidomastoid

The scalene muscles are located deep in relation to the SCM muscle and lateral to the cervical spine, connecting the vertebrae to the first two ribs. They can be thought of as having three distinct parts: anterior, middle and posterior. They play the role of accessory breathing muscles but are also involved in lateral flexion and flexion of the neck and maintaining the static position of the head and neck.

Trapezius and levator scapulae are some of the other important muscles that are located in the region of the neck. We will explore these in more detail in the next chapter on the shoulder.

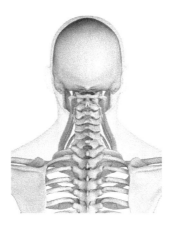

Part of the middle scalenes

Nerves, blood vessels and lymphatics

Many important blood vessels, nerves and lymphatic vessels pass through the region of the neck.

Cervical nerves are spinal nerves that arise from the cervical region of the spinal cord. There are eight pairs of cervical nerves, denoted C1 to C8. Shortly after branching out of the spinal cord, the cervical nerves form the cervical and brachial plexuses that then give rise to peripheral nerves that maintain a significant motor function in the head, neck, upper limbs and diaphragm, as well as sensation in the head, neck, shoulders and upper limbs.

The common carotid artery travels up the neck and divides into the internal and external carotid arteries. The internal carotid artery then enters the cranium through the carotid canal in the temporal bone. The anterior brain region is supplied by the internal carotid arteries and the posterior circulation is fed by the vertebral arteries. The vertebral arteries arise from the subclavian arteries and ascend through the cervical vertebrae via the transverse foramina. They enter the cranium through the foramen of the occipital bone. The vertebral arteries supply the cerebellum, brain stem and underside of the cerebrum.

The head and neck contain a rich and elaborate lymphatic network of more than 300 nodes and their intermediate channels, bound together with the muscles, nerves and vessels of this region (Koroulakis and

Agarwal 2019). This lymphatic drainage originates at the base of the skull and then proceeds to the jugular chain adjacent to the internal jugular vein.

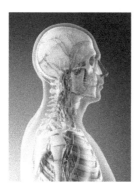

Neck vessels

Common cervical spine injuries and conditions

In this section we will explore some of the most common cervical spine injuries and conditions that affect our population.

Neck pain

Lifetime prevalence of neck pain has been reported to be 26–71% with 12-month prevalence estimates ranging from 30% to 50%. Most people (50–85%) in the general population with neck pain do not experience a complete resolution of this problem (Hogg-Johnson *et al.* 2008). Neck pain has been reported to account for approximately 15% of hospital physiotherapy and 30% of chiropractic visits (Benyamin *et al.* 2009). Similar to back pain, most cases of acute (less than six weeks' duration) neck pain will resolve to a large extent within two months, but close to 50% of patients will continue to have some pain or frequent recurrences one year after the original occurrence (Vasseljen *et al.* 2013).

Very little is known about the causes of neck pain. The epidemiologic studies do not reveal either the source or the cause of pain. A literature review by Hogg-Johnson *et al.* (2008) suggested that modifiable factors for neck pain include smoking, exposure to tobacco and psychological health. They did not identify intervertebral disc degeneration as a risk factor.

A literature review by Carroll *et al.* (2008) reported that better psychologic health, greater optimism and greater social support predicted a better outcome in primary care and general population samples with initial neck pain. Poor psychologic health and worrying, becoming angry or becoming frustrated in response to neck pain were associated with poorer prognosis.

Although certain occupations such as office and computer workers, manual laborers and healthcare workers have been found in some studies to have a higher incidence of neck pain, the major workplace factors associated with the condition are low job satisfaction and perceived poor workplace environment (Côté *et al.* 2009).

Cervical disc herniation and radiculopathy

We have discussed disc herniation in Chapter 6. Cervical radiculopathy is a clinical condition resulting from compression of cervical nerve roots. The clinical manifestations of cervical radiculopathy are broad and may include pain, sensory deficits, motor deficits, diminished reflexes or any combination of the above. Research into cervical disc herniation and radiculopathy is not as extensive as that of similar lumbar spine conditions.

The cause of cervical spine disc herniations is not clearly understood and is thought to be multifactorial. The proposed risk factors include male gender, smoking, heavy lifting, frequent diving from a board and occupation. Preliminary evidence suggests the incidence of cervical disc herniations is higher in army aviators, professional drivers and those who operate vibrating equipment (Wong *et al.* 2014). However, one study reported only 15% of cases had a history of physical exertion or trauma preceding the onset of symptoms (Radhakrishnan *et al.* 1994). Kelsey *et al.* (1984) reported that up to 30% of patients report the onset of pain when sitting, walking or standing.

The systematic review by Iyer and Kim (2016) suggested that the majority of cases of cervical radiculopathy are not due to disc herniation, but rather due to cervical spondylosis (degenerative disc disease) where the breakdown of the disc with age leads to decreased disc height and narrowing of the foramen.

A systematic review of the literature on symptomatic cervical disc herniation with radiculopathy by Wong *et al.* (2014) reported that most patients experience substantial improvements within four to six months post-onset. They noted that the time to complete recovery ranged from 24 to 36 months in most patients.

Thoracic outlet syndrome (TOS)

TOS is a term used to describe a group of disorders that occur when there is compression, injury or irritation of the nerves (neurogenic TOS) and/ or blood vessels (vascular TOS) in the lower neck and upper chest area. TOS is named for the space between the lower neck and upper chest (the thoracic outlet) where this grouping of nerves and blood vessels is found. Patients present with symptoms and signs of arterial insufficiency, venous obstruction, painless wasting of intrinsic hand muscles, paresthesia (burning or prickling sensation) and pain.

Reported incidences of TOS range from 0.3% to 8% of the population. TOS is more commonly observed in women, and the onset of symptoms usually occurs between 20 and 50 years of age (Huang and Zager 2004).

According to Sanders, Hammond and Rao (2007), 90% of TOS patients have neurogenic TOS. They stated that vascular TOS is almost always associated with a cervical rib, which is an additional rib that arises from the seventh cervical vertebra. Cervical ribs are thought to occur in less than 1% of the population and are more common in women (Brewin, Hill and Ellis 2009). Most cervical ribs do not produce symptoms.

Cervical stenosis

Cervical stenosis is a narrowing of the spinal canal. Facet-joint degenerative changes can result in enlargement of these small joints, which, in association with thickening of the ligamentum flavum, can contribute to canal stenosis. In some cases, the narrowing can put pressure on the spinal cord.

Lee, Cassinelli and Riew (2007) estimated that cervical stenosis is present in nearly 5% of the adult population, approximately 7% of the population who are 50 years of age or older and 9% of the population who are 70 years of age or older.

In a landmark study, Boden *et al.* (1990) reported that 19% of patients with no symptoms had abnormal findings on scans of their cervical spine and that the prevalence increased with age.

Of these asymptomatic subjects who were younger than 40 years of age, 10% had a herniated disc and 4% had cervical stenosis. Of the subjects who were older than 40 years of age, 5% had a herniated disc, 3% had bulging of the disc and 20% had cervical stenosis. Narrowing of a disc space, degeneration of a disc, bone spurs or compression of the cord were also recorded. The disc was degenerated or narrowed at one level or more in 25% of the subjects who were younger than 40 years of age and in almost 60% of those who were older than 40 years of age.

INTELLIGENT MOVEMENT PRINCIPLE – NO NATURAL MOVEMENT IS INHERENTLY BAD

There are many movements that are regularly condemned in the yoga world. There appears to be widespread belief that we should never lock our knees or elbows, that internally rotating our shoulders in Downward Facing Dog (Adho Mukha Svanasana) is bad, that flexing the spine is harmful, that the knee should never move beyond the ankle in a High Lunge and that we should never roll our heads in a full circle, to mention just a few. These are all in fact natural movements that our body is designed to make and no inherent harm is to be done from making these movements as long as we follow a few simple guidelines: that we are aware of the movement that we are making, that we have full control over the range of the movement, that there is no pain elicited as a result of the movement and that the movement is accompanied by adequate breath.

So, to relate this specifically to the head and neck, while rolling the head in a circle or taking the neck into extension doesn't feel great for everyone, these are not inherently bad movements. Again, the key is to move slowly, with awareness and control, and to stay within a pain-free range.

It is worth noting that the cervical canal diameter is decreased with extension of the neck (Zeng *et al.* 2016) and therefore a degree of caution may need to be taken here with students who have symptoms of cervical stenosis.

Later in the chapter we will address how important it is to mobilize the neck in order for it to remain healthy and functional.

Forward head posture (FHP)

FHP, commonly known as 'text-neck', is often cited as being one of the leading causes of neck pain, although the little research that has explored this relationship is inconclusive. A recent study by Damasceno *et al.* (2018) did not show an association between 'text-neck' and neck pain in young adults aged 18–21. A systematic review and meta-analysis by Sheikhhoseini *et al.* (2018) reported that the precise nature of the relationship between FHP and musculoskeletal pain remains to be established. Interestingly, a small study by Koseki *et al.* (2019) reported that FHP causes expansion of the upper thorax and contraction of the lower thorax, and the authors noted that these changes cause decreased respiratory function.

My take on this controversial topic is that it may be a more efficient use of our time and energy to focus on mobilizing the head and neck regularly instead of focusing on our static head and neck posture. A study by Kim, Kim and Son (2018) found that the occurrence of cervical area pain was higher amongst subjects who had a decreased CVJ motion.

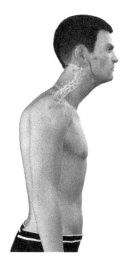

Forward head posture

Key yoga asanas and how to adapt them

We will now explore some asanas that may present a challenge to students who are affected by the common injuries or conditions that we have discussed above and look at some of the ways that these can be adapted in order to make them more accessible.

Backbends

While maintaining the range of movement of the head and neck is very important, in asanas such as Camel Pose (Ustrasana) and Upward Facing Dog (Urdhva Mukha Svanasana) it can often feel more supportive to either keep the cervical spine in a more neutral position or even gently lower the chin towards the chest. When choosing to extend the neck here it is important to do this slowly and with control. It is best to avoid 'dropping the head back' without full control of the range of extension. Depressing the shoulder girdle (drawing the shoulder blades down) can also help in these asanas by maintaining space between the occiput and the shoulders.

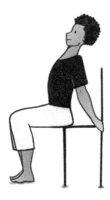

Camel Pose

Supported Shoulderstand

Supported Shoulderstand (Salamba Sarvangasana) should be thought of as an arm-balance and it is important that the back of the neck (including the spinous process of C7) is not in contact with the mat and therefore bearing weight. Use a blanket to raise the shoulders slightly higher than the back of the head and gently retract the shoulder girdles (drawing the shoulder blades towards each other).

It is important to note that Supported Shoulderstand is not accessible for many students. Great alternatives to this asana, that provide similar benefits associated with inverting the body, include Legs-Up-The-Wall (Viparita Karani) and Supported Bridge Pose (Setu Bandha Sarvangasana). In each of these poses the pelvis can be placed on a bolster.

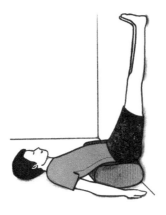

Legs-Up-The-Wall

Headstand

Headstand (Sirsasana) is another arm-balance that is not accessible for most students. It is important that the great majority of the weight of the body is not supported by the head or neck in this asana, which requires significant upper limb strength and coordination. Half Headstand, where the students walk their feet forward until their hips are roughly above their shoulders, can be a good alternative for some. Headstand can also be practiced by supporting the shoulders with two stacks of foam blocks that are slightly taller than the height of the head and neck. These stacks should be placed against a wall and, similar to Half Headstand, one can then walk the feet forward until the hips are above the shoulders. Two sturdy chairs pressed against a wall and facing each other can also be used as the support here, with blankets to add some cushioning for the shoulders.

Triangle Pose

In Extended Triangle Pose (Trikonasana) it is important to turn the head in whichever direction feels most comfortable for the neck. Holding the head so that it is in line with the spine can be challenging for many students. There is always the option to gently lower the head down towards the supporting shoulder.

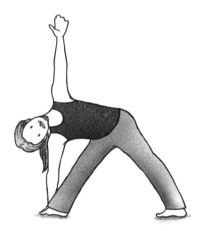

Extended Triangle Pose with lateral neck flexion

Twists

In asanas that involve rotation of the spine it can be tempting to lead the movement with the head and neck, since this region has the greatest amount of rotational range of movement in the spine. Try to keep the chin in line with the breastbone as you rotate the thoracic spine. Then you have the option to slowly turn the head in the direction of the twist.

Improving the overall health of the cervical spine

This section addresses some effective ways in which we can improve and maintain the health and functioning of our cervical spine. It is intended to be a general guide for yoga practitioners and teachers and is not a replacement for the personal advice of a health professional.

Cervical spine mobility

Cohen (2015) stated that cervical and scapular stretching and strengthening exercises have been found to provide intermediate-term relief for mechanical neck pain. As we discussed earlier, it is important to move slowly and with control and to stay within pain-free range of movement. You always have the option to decrease the size of the movements or to rest at any time.

EXERCISE ONE

1. Place one hand on your breastbone to stabilize your thoracic spine.

2. Slowly shift your head forward and back in the horizontal plane, without lowering or lifting your chin.

3. After a few repetitions rest back in a neutral position.

4. Now place your index fingers directly in front of your eyes.

5. Without rotating your head side to side, slowly shift your head to the right and then to the left in the horizontal plane.

6. After a few repetitions rest back in a neutral position.

Placing your index fingers in front of your eyes helps you to stabilize your upper body while you focus on isolating just your neck movements. These movements may feel a little strange and staggered at first but with practice they will quickly become smoother and more controlled.

We will now combine all four of these movements.

1. Place your hand back onto your breastbone.

2. Slowly shift your head forward, to the right, back and to the left.

3. Repeat this for a few cycles and then repeat this in the opposite direction.

4. Rest and take a few moments to notice how your neck is feeling.

EXERCISE TWO

1. Slowly lower your chin towards your chest and then gently lift your chin up.

2. Repeat this slowly for a few cycles.

3. Slowly turn your head to the right and then to the left for a few repetitions.

4. Gently lower one ear down towards your shoulder on that side.

5. Control your head back to the center and then repeat on the opposite side.

6. Repeat this for a few cycles noticing how one side feels compared to the other.

7. You can lower your chin down towards your breastbone and gently roll your head side to side.

8. You can also lift your chin slightly and roll your head slightly side to side.

9. You now have the option to combine all of these movements by slowly moving your head around in a circle.

10. Repeat this in the opposite direction.

Releasing jaw tension

I mentioned earlier that it has been suggested that cranio-cervical posture is significantly influenced by the TMJ (An *et al.* 2015). Gently massaging the TMJ with the fingertips can help to develop our awareness of this significant area and potentially reduce tension here. The following movements are a great way to develop more control over the TMJ and will also potentially help to reduce unwanted tension over time. Try to open your mouth as wide as possible while making the movement as slow as possible. Now close your mouth as slowly as possible. Repeat this a couple of times throughout the day.

Focusing on abdominal breathing

The term 'chest breathing' describes the action of breathing predominantly into the upper chest region and involves the action of the accessory muscles of respiration (including the sternocleidomastoids, scalenes and levator scapulae). When we primarily breathe in this way the accessory muscles can become overused and tight, potentially impacting the health and function of the cervical spine. 'Abdominal breathing' involves drawing our focus downwards towards the lower ribs and abdomen as we breathe, involving less action by the accessory muscles.

Thoracic spine mobility

All of the practices that we explored in the previous chapter to improve the health and function of the thoracic spine will also have a positive impact on the cervical spine.

Shoulder girdle and shoulder joint mobility

In the next chapter we will explore ways to improve the health and function of the shoulder girdle and shoulder joint. All of these practices will also have a positive impact on the cervical spine.

A systematic review by Gross *et al.* (2015) reported that the use of strengthening and endurance exercises for the cervico-scapulo-thoracic region and shoulder may be beneficial in reducing pain and improving function in the neck. However, the review states that when only stretching exercises were used no beneficial effects may be expected.

Part 3

THE UPPER LIMB

A free online class incorporating most of the practices described in this part can be found at https://lddy.no/pat7.

Chapter 9

THE SHOULDER

The shoulder complex is the region where the upper limb connects to the axial skeleton and is made up of three bones: the upper arm bone (humerus), the shoulder blade (scapula) and the collarbone (clavicle). The relationship between these three bones creates a huge range of movement for the upper limb; the main function being to position the hand to affect functional activities. The 'scapulohumeral rhythm' first described by Codman (1934) is the pattern of muscle contractions and motion that occurs between the scapula and the humerus. While these areas are designed to work seamlessly together, we will explore them separately in an attempt to really understand the anatomy and function of each element.

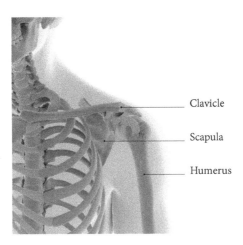

Clavicle

Scapula

Humerus

Shoulder complex

The anatomy of the shoulder girdle

The shoulder girdle is made up of the clavicle and the scapula which articulate to form a cage-like structure that sits on the side of the ribcage and connects the upper limb to the axial skeleton.

The clavicle

The clavicle forms the anterior portion of the shoulder girdle. It is a long, double-curved bone that lies horizontally, immediately above the first rib. It articulates medially with the manubrium of the sternum to form the sternoclavicular joint, and laterally with the acromion of the scapula to form the acromioclavicular joint.

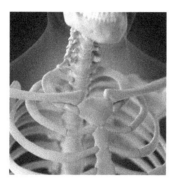

Sternoclavicular joints

The scapula

The scapula is a triangular, flat bone that forms the posterior of the shoulder girdle and serves as a site for attachment for many muscles. It provides a stable base from which shoulder joint mobility occurs (Voight and Thomson 2000).

The posterior surface of the scapula is subdivided into two unequal parts by the 'spine' of the scapula, which is a prominent plate of bone that crosses the upper part of the scapula obliquely.

Originating from the superolateral surface of the anterior scapula (the side facing the ribcage) is the coracoid process. It is a hook-like projection, which lies just underneath the clavicle and serves as the attachment site for pectoralis minor and the short head of biceps brachii.

The acromion forms the summit of the shoulder complex, and is a large, somewhat oblong process, projecting at first laterally, and then curving forward and upward, so as to overhang the glenoid cavity of the shoulder joint. The acromioclavicular joint connects the clavicle to the acromion.

On the lateral surface of the scapula is the glenoid fossa, a shallow cavity that articulates with the head of the humerus to form the gleno-humeral (shoulder) joint.

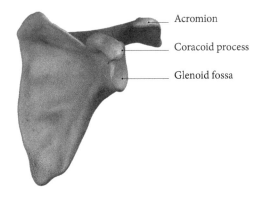

Acromion

Coracoid process

Glenoid fossa

Anterior view of left scapula

There are no bony attachments, ligaments or tendons that connect the scapula to the ribcage. A suction mechanism is provided by the muscular attachments of the serratus anterior and subscapularis which holds the scapula in close proximity to the thorax and allows it to glide over the rib-cage (Peat 1986). This greatly enhances the range of movement of the shoulder girdle and consequently the upper limb.

Stability of the scapulo-thoracic region therefore depends on coordinated activity of the surrounding musculature. This also means that the only bone-to-bone connection between the upper limb and the axial skeleton is the small sternoclavicular joint. When we bear weight on the upper limbs it is therefore important to have sufficient awareness, control and strength in the muscles of the shoulder girdle to ensure that the load is shared across the whole shoulder complex and not just focused on the shoulder joint, sternoclavicular joint and acromioclavicular joint.

Movements of the shoulder girdle

We will now explore six main movements of the shoulder girdle.

Elevation is moving the shoulder girdle up towards the ear, while depression is moving the shoulder girdle down away from the ear. Later in the chapter we will explore why these are both equally important movements.

Protraction is drawing the scapula away from the midline of the body. In full scapular protraction the scapula follows the contour of the ribs which results in the glenoid fossa facing anteriorly with the full scapula in contact with the ribcage (Levangie and Norkin 2005). Protraction tends to be coupled with a degree of thoracic flexion.

Retraction is moving the scapula towards the midline of the body and tends to be coupled with thoracic extension.

Upward rotation describes a swinging movement roughly in the frontal plane whereby the lower tip of the scapula moves in a superolateral direction away from the midline. In a neutral scapular position, the glenoid fossa faces laterally, but as the scapula begins to upwardly rotate the glenoid fossa begins to face upwards. This plays a significant role in increasing the range of movement of the arm overhead. This motion also places the glenoid fossa in a position to support and stabilize the head of the raised humerus (Neumann 2009). According to Levangie and Norkin (2005) the shoulder girdle is able to upwardly rotate 60°.

Downward rotation describes the swinging movement, again roughly in the frontal plane, whereby the lower tip of the scapula moves in an inferomedial direction towards the midline.

Downward rotation of the scapula occurs as the arm is returned to the side from a raised position. The movement usually ends when the scapula has returned to its anatomical or neutral position (Neumann 2009).

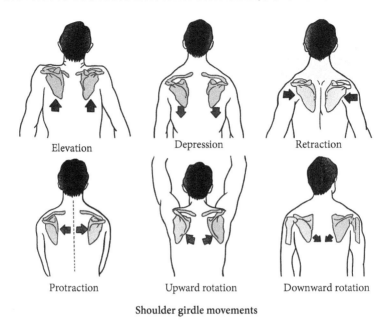

Elevation

Depression

Retraction

Protraction

Upward rotation

Downward rotation

Shoulder girdle movements

The musculature of the shoulder girdle

Pectoralis minor originates from the third, fourth and fifth ribs and inserts on the coracoid process of the scapula. It lies beneath pectoralis major and is involved in depression, protraction and downward rotation of the scapula.

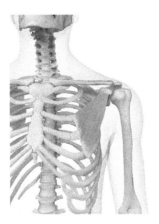

Pectoralis minor

Serratus anterior originates from the upper nine ribs and inserts on the medial border of the scapula from the inside. It forms the lateral part of the chest wall and prevents winging of the scapulae (which we will discuss later in the chapter). It is involved in protraction and some upward rotation of the scapula.

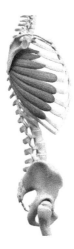

Serratus anterior

Levator scapula originates from the first four cervical vertebrae, inserts on the superior aspect of the scapula and is involved in elevation of the scapulae. The muscle also assists in downward rotation of the shoulder girdle.

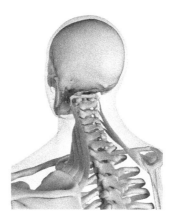

Levator scapulae

Rhomboid major and minor are flat, rectangular muscles that originate from the spinous processes of the vertebrae and insert on the medial border of the scapula. They are involved in retraction and downward rotation of the scapula.

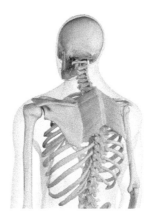

Rhomboids

Trapezius is a huge muscle that originates at the base of the skull and the spinous processes of C2 through T12. It inserts on the clavicle and the spine of the scapula. The upper fibers elevate the shoulder girdle while the lower fibers depress the shoulder girdle.

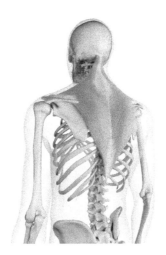

Trapezius

WHY IS DEPRESSION OF THE SHOULDER GIRDLES SUCH A POPULAR CUE IN YOGA?

In the wider yoga community, there tends to be a preference for drawing the shoulder blades down in almost every asana and often a belief that this is 'right' and that lifting the shoulder blades towards the ears is 'wrong'. As we have just described, the anatomical term for lifting the shoulder blades is elevation and the main muscle creating this movement is trapezius (upper fibers).

Keeping the shoulder blades elevated throughout an asana can make it more challenging to breathe fully, but I sense that the aversion to active elevation amongst many teachers stems from a deeper misconception that this action will strengthen the upper fibers of the trapezius, therefore shortening the muscle and creating further tightness in this region. We explored this specific topic earlier in the handbook and discussed how strengthening does not lead to shortening of muscle tissue and can often be a helpful way to decrease perceived muscle tightness.

Depressing the shoulder girdles is not a bad thing to do, but if we also add active shoulder girdle elevation into our regular movement routine, we'll most likely notice a decrease in upper trapezius tightness, and we'll be increasing our overall shoulder girdle mobility.

The anatomy of the shoulder joint

Also known as the glenohumeral joint, the shoulder joint is a ball-and-socket joint that involves the articulation between the head of the humerus and the shallow glenoid fossa of the scapula. The shoulder joint has the greatest mobility of all our joints, but it is therefore the least stable joint in the body.

The ligaments of the shoulder joint limit the amount of movement made by the joint, but they do not maintain the contact of the articulating surfaces. The joint capsule is so remarkably loose and lax that it also has no action in keeping the humerus and glenoid fossa in contact (Gray *et al.* 2005). It is mainly the role of the 'rotator cuff' muscles to provide the majority of the joint stability.

The glenoid labrum is a fibrocartilaginous ring that is thought to provide additional depth to the glenoid fossa and protect the edges of the bone (Gray *et al.* 2005). The joint is also stabilized above by an arch, formed by the coracoid process, the acromion and the coracoacromial ligament.

The shoulder joint is capable of every variety of movement: flexion and extension, abduction and adduction, and external and internal rotation.

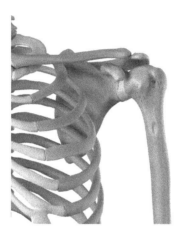

Shoulder joint

The shoulder joint musculature

Deltoid has three parts that originate from the clavicle, acromion and scapulae respectively and insert on the lateral humerus. The anterior deltoid is involved in horizontal adduction, flexion and internal rotation of the shoulder joint. The lateral deltoid is involved in shoulder joint abduction, while the posterior deltoid is involved in shoulder joint extension.

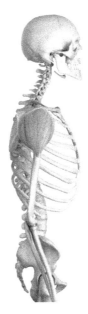

Deltoid

Pectoralis major forms a significant part of the front of the chest, originating from the clavicle and the sternum and inserting on the inside of the proximal humerus. It is involved in adduction, internal rotation and flexion from a position of hyperextension (when the arm is behind the torso).

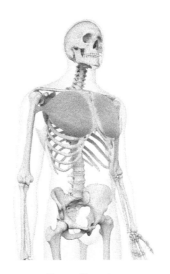

Pectoralis major

Latissimus dorsi makes up two-thirds of the superficial back muscles. It has a huge origin at the iliac crest, on the spinous processes of the lower half of the vertebrae, the lower three ribs and the inferior scapula. It has a tiny insertion on the proximal humerus and is involved in adduction, extension and internal rotation of the shoulder joint.

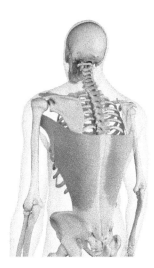

Latissimus dorsi

The 'rotator cuff' is a set of four muscles that stabilize the humeral head in the glenoid fossa and are also involved in specific shoulder joint movements. Infraspinatus lies below the spine of the scapula and inserts on the greater tuberosity of the humerus. It works alongside teres minor to produce external rotation. Supraspinatus lies above the spine of the scapula and also inserts on the greater tuberosity of the humerus and initiates arm abduction. Subscapularis lies beneath the scapula, inserts on the lesser tuberosity of the humeral head and is involved in internal rotation.

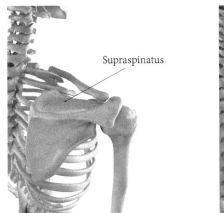
Supraspinatus

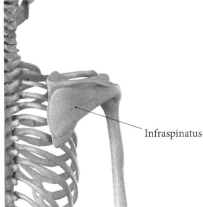
Infraspinatus

It is interesting to note that in terms of external rotation, only infraspinatus and teres minor are involved. In terms of internal rotation, anterior deltoid, latissimus dorsi, pectoralis major and subscapularis are all involved.

We have focused on the role muscles have on shoulder joint and shoulder girdle movement when the spine is fixed. It is important to note that when the upper limbs are fixed these muscles will act to move the spine; for example, latissimus dorsi will extend the spine.

Common shoulder injuries and conditions

In this section we will explore some of the most common shoulder injuries and conditions that affect our population.

Subacromial impingement syndrome (SIS)

The term SIS encompasses shoulder pain and pathology originating from the tendon or bursa in the subacromial space. This condition is well recognized clinically, presenting as anterolateral shoulder pain experienced when the arm is elevated. SIS and rotator cuff tendinopathy are considered to be the most common causes of shoulder pain. The proportion of the population that are believed to have this condition at any given time has been estimated to be between 2.4% and 14% (Littlewood, May and Walters 2013).

The cause of SIS is still not fully understood and is based on a hypothesis that acromial irritation leads to external abrasion of the bursa and rotator cuff. Neer (1972) argued that this occurs principally in flexion of the shoulder joint and described a clinical test, the '(Neer) impingement sign', to reproduce the associated symptoms. The test involves restricting scapular movement and forcing the arm into flexion while the shoulder joint remains internally rotated (Neer 1983). According to Neer, this maneuver causes the greater tuberosity of the humerus to impinge against the acromion. He argued that 95% of rotator cuff tears are initiated by impingement and that trauma may enlarge a tear but is rarely the principal factor. Neer also stated that the reason rotator cuff tears develop in some people and not others is principally due to the shape of the acromion.

However, surgery aiming to remove the cause of the impingement irritation (i.e., the acromion) is no more clinically effective than a structured rehabilitation program (Ketola, Lehtinen and Arnala 2017). There is little evidence for an acromial impingement model, and it has been suggested that a more appropriate name for this condition is 'subacromial pain syndrome' (Lewis 2011).

CURRENT THOUGHTS ON PERSISTENT PAIN

Pain and tissue damage do not always correlate. It is very possible to have tissue damage without experiencing pain and it is also possible to experience pain when there is no apparent tissue damage. Pretty much every assumed dysfunction that is discussed (posture, tightness, weakness, degeneration) can exist in people without pain. Pain tells us that there is a problem, but it rarely tells us what the problem is, where it is or how bad it is.

Pain can often be correlated with depression, fear, rumination and worries about injury. Recent studies have provided incontrovertible evidence that psychopathology and other psychosocial factors can influence both the development of persistent pain conditions and the response to treatment. In a study by Polatin *et al.* (1993) conducted with 200 patients who had persistent lower back pain (LBP), the authors found that 77% met lifetime criteria and 59% demonstrated current symptoms for at least one psychiatric diagnosis, with the most common being depression, substance abuse and anxiety disorders. Notably, more than 50% of those with depression and more than 90% of patients with substance abuse or an anxiety disorder experienced symptoms before the onset of LBP. Most, but not all, studies have shown untreated psychopathology to negatively affect LBP treatment outcomes (Fayad *et al.* 2004). This does not mean that pain is 'all in one's head'. It means that there is often a strong link between experiencing pain and one's mental resilience.

Social factors have also been demonstrated to impact the prognosis of LBP. These include return-to-work issues, catastrophizing, poor role models, codependency behavior, inadequate coping mechanisms and attitudes, beliefs and expectations (Seres 2003). To optimize outcomes, the identification and treatment of associated psychosocial issues is of paramount importance. This is best accomplished via a multidisciplinary approach. The biopsychosocial model is therefore very important when trying to address persistent pain.

Experiencing some pain at different stages of our lives is a normal part of being human. It is our response to the pain that tends to be most significant. Often understanding and acknowledging pain can be desensitizing.

In the introduction to this book I described how 'an injury essentially occurs when the load applied to a region of the body exceeds that region's ability to withstand such a load'. Pain could be thought about in a similar way: all the mechanical loads and all the emotional stressors in your life exceeding your perceived ability to withstand or adapt to these.

Rotator cuff tears

Tears in the rotator cuff muscles and tendons are common and incidence increases with age. Approximately 54% of adults older than 60 years have a partial or complete rotator cuff tear, compared with only 4% of those aged 40–60 years (Bartolozzi, Andreychik and Ahmad 1994). Symptoms include pain, weakness and limitation of shoulder joint motion.

Yamamoto *et al.* (2010) reported that 17% of subjects without shoulder symptoms had rotator cuff tears. A systematic review by Teunis *et al.* (2014) stated that the prevalence of rotator cuff abnormalities in asymptomatic people is high enough for degeneration of the rotator cuff to be considered a common aspect of normal human aging and makes it difficult to determine when an abnormality is new (e.g., after a dislocation) or is the cause of symptoms.

Epidemiological data on the association between mechanical overuse and cuff tearing are inconclusive but an association has been found with smoking (Sambandam *et al.* 2015). Scapular instability is found in as many as 68% of cases of rotator cuff problems and 100% of glenohumeral instability problems (Paine and Voight 2013).

Frozen shoulder (adhesive capsulitis)

Adhesive capsulitis describes a pathological process in which the body forms excessive scar tissue or adhesions across the glenohumeral joint, leading to pain, stiffness and dysfunction. It is a condition that can occur spontaneously or following shoulder surgery or trauma (Neviaser and Neviaser 2011). Codman (1934) coined the term 'frozen shoulder' to emphasize the debilitating loss of shoulder motion in patients afflicted with this condition. It is now generally accepted that the development of adhesive capsulitis involves an inflammatory as well as fibrotic process (Le *et al.* 2017).

The incidence of adhesive capsulitis in the general population is approximately 3–5% but is as high as 20% in patients with diabetes (Le *et al.* 2017). Idiopathic (unknown cause) adhesive capsulitis often involves the nondominant arm, although bilateral involvement has been reported in up to 40–50% of cases (Manske and Prohaska 2008). It is estimated that 70% of patients with adhesive shoulder capsulitis are women (Sheridan and Hannafin 2006). Demographic studies have shown that most patients with adhesive capsulitis (84%) fall within the age range of 40–59 years (Boyle-Walker *et al.* 1997).

In a review by Le *et al.* (2017) the authors stated that adhesive capsulitis is often regarded as a self-limiting disease that resolves in one to three years. However, the authors note that various studies have shown that between 20% and 50% of patients may go on to develop long-lasting symptoms.

Winged scapula

The term 'winged scapula' is used when the muscles of the scapula are too weak, resulting in a limited ability to stabilize the scapula. As a result, the medial or lateral border of the scapula protrudes like wings. Scapular winging is one of the most common abnormalities of the scapulo-thoracic articulation. Winged scapula can have a neurological or a musculoskeletal cause.

When the scapula fails to perform its stabilization role the function of the shoulder complex becomes inefficient, which can not only result in decreased neuromuscular performance but also may predispose the individual to injury of the glenohumeral joint. Loss of serratus anterior function results in reductions in both glenohumeral flexion and abduction (Kamkar, Irrgang and Whitney 1993).

Shoulder dislocation (glenohumeral subluxation)

The shoulder is the most commonly dislocated large joint (Yang *et al.* 2011) due to the fact that it has the largest range of movement of any joint in the body. The majority of dislocations occur in men aged under 40 years and most are sports injuries. After a first-time traumatic shoulder dislocation, approximately 50% of people develop recurrent shoulder dislocation within two years (Kavaja *et al.* 2018).

Key yoga asanas and how to adapt them

We will now explore some asanas that may present a challenge to students who are affected by the common injuries or conditions that we have discussed above and look at some of the ways that these can be adapted in order to make them more accessible.

Standing asanas

In any standing asana where the arms are typically required to reach up in front or out to the sides of the body, it is always helpful to invite students to lift their arms as far as is comfortable with the options to rest their hands on their hips or cross their arms over their shoulders.

Binding can also create quite the challenge. In Eagle Pose (Garudasana) options include crossing one's arms in front of the chest or crossing the arms at the elbows but keeping the hands separated.

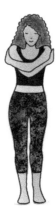

Eagle Pose arm variations

A yoga strap is a really helpful prop when shoulder mobility is limited. A good example is in Dancer Pose (Natarajasana) where a strap can be placed over the back foot and then looped over the top of the shoulder.

Downward Facing Dog (Adho Mukha Svanasana)

Have you ever asked your students to 'rest in Downward Dog' or heard another teacher say this? Downward Facing Dog (Adho Mukha Svanasana) can be a very challenging asana for many students, particularly those who are working with a shoulder injury or condition. Thankfully, there are many different ways that we can practice the asana so that it can be more accessible.

Raising the level of the hands shifts the center of gravity back and takes a little pressure off the upper limbs. You can place foam blocks under your hands or even support your hands on a sturdy chair.

Downward Facing Dog can be practiced against a wall. Stand facing the wall with your arms reaching forward and a short space between the wall and your fingertips. Inhale as you slowly lift your arms to a comfortable height, and as you exhale fold at your hips, press your pelvis back and place your hands on the wall. Adjust the position of your feet and hands as needed.

For the many students who struggle to place their heels on the floor there is the option to practice facing away from the wall and pressing the heels into the wall for support. Foam blocks can also be positioned under the heels to offer a greater sense of grounding.

Puppy Pose (Uttana Shishosana) is another great variation. Lower your knees to the ground and keep your thighs vertical as you reach your hands forward. A more restorative version of the asana is to rest your forehead on a bolster or a pile of stacked blankets, and this can also take some of the load out of the shoulders.

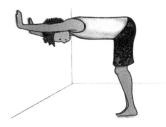

Downward Facing Dog

Four Limbed Staff Pose (Chaturanga Dandasana)

Chaturanga is another very common asana that when taught in the 'traditional' way is not accessible to many students. Again, there are many creative ways to adapt the asana in order to make it much more accessible.

Chaturanga can be practiced against a wall. Stand facing the wall with your hands pressing into the wall, roughly at shoulder-height and slightly wider than your shoulders. Slowly begin to bend at the elbows as you lift up onto the balls of your feet and lower your chest and chin down towards the wall.

Chaturanga can also be practiced at home on an incline against the kitchen counter. Another good variation is to place foam blocks under your hands and lower your knees to the mat before bending at the elbows.

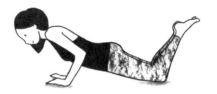

Four Limbed Staff Pose

Plank Pose (Kumbhakasana)

A more accessible variation of Plank Pose (Kumbhakasana) can be practiced by lowering your forearms to the mat with your elbows under your shoulders. Your knees can also be lowered; ensure you keep them behind your hips.

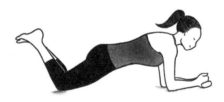

Plank Pose

Improving the overall health of the shoulder

This section addresses some effective ways in which we can all improve and maintain the health and functioning of our shoulders. It is intended to be a general guide for yoga practitioners and teachers and is not a replacement for the personal advice of a health professional.

Shoulder girdle mobility

Start in a comfortable seated position where you can easily find a neutral position throughout the length of your spine.

1. Gently brace your abdomen so that your spine remains in this position and reach your arms forward.

2. You can always squeeze a foam block between your hands too.

3. Slowly lift your scapulae up towards your ears.

4. Keep them elevated as you draw them together into retraction.

5. Keep this position of retraction as you slowly draw your scapulae down.

6. Now draw them apart into protraction.

7. Rest for a moment and then repeat this in the opposite direction: retracting, then elevating, then protracting and finally depressing your scapulae.

On the next cycle you can start to add some internal resistance by imaging that there is a force trying to prevent you from moving in each direction. You can also practice holding a foam block or wooden brick between your hands. Notice the stages that feel particularly challenging or particularly stiff or tight.

This exercise can also be practiced on your back using the floor to provide feedback. The retraction and protraction movements can be practiced with the palms of your hands pressing into a wall and your hands placed roughly shoulder-width and shoulder-height. Keep your abdomen gently braced and your arms straight.

Once you have become more familiar with this exercise and feel ready to increase the intensity there is the option to repeat it on your hands and knees. This position increases the load applied to the shoulder complex and makes each movement significantly more challenging. You can then begin to step your knees further and further back until you are eventually in Plank Pose. You can also keep your knees under your hips, hover your knees an inch off the mat and repeat the exercise. Take your time and be patient about progressing to these steps. If you have increased the intensity too quickly, rest and take things down a notch.

Active internal rotation

In my experience there tend to be few opportunities to actively internally rotate the shoulder joints in a traditional yoga practice. We mainly use internal rotation to help us to bind and then focus on external rotation.

1. In a comfortable seated position, imagine that you are holding on to two large light bulbs.

2. Keep your arms straight and, focusing the movement at the shoulder joint, slowly screw the light bulbs in and out. It can help to focus on the armpits turning to face each other and then turning away from each other.

3. Now change the position of your arms with the option of creating fists with your hands. You can reach them forward, up, back or to the sides. There is an infinite number of possible positions here.

4. Make the movements slow and controlled and stay within a pain-free range.

You can also explore active internal and external rotation in Puppy Pose (Uttana Shishosana), in Child's Pose (Balasana), on your hands and knees or in Downward Facing Dog (Adho Mukha Svanasana). Build up the intensity slowly.

Active extension

There also tend to be few opportunities to actively extend the shoulder joints in a traditional yoga practice. We move our arms behind our torso quite regularly but so often prop them there by clasping our hands together or using the support of the floor or a yoga strap.

1. Back in your comfortable seated position, reach both of your arms out to the side.

2. Bend your elbows and place your hands either behind your neck or on your shoulders.

3. Keep your elbows where they are.

4.   Slowly straighten and bend one arm at a time. You can then straighten and bend both arms together.

5.   Notice the work being done to keep your shoulders in this position.

Rest your arms by your sides for a moment and when you're ready try this exercise.

1.   Gently brace your abdomen so that the movements are focused on the shoulder joints.

2.   Keep your elbows straight and slowly lift your arms back behind you, as if you are doing a seated reverse Plank Pose.

3.   Resist the temptation to clasp your hands together but imagine that you are squeezing a block between your hands.

4.   After a few breaths, lower your arms and rest.

5.   Repeat the exercise as desired.

Isolating shoulder joint movement

As we have discussed earlier in this chapter, the whole shoulder complex is designed to work seamlessly together. However, it is also beneficial to train ourselves to isolate shoulder joint movements from those of the shoulder girdle and thoracic spine.

The following exercise focuses on isolating shoulder joint movements from shoulder girdle movements.

1.   Find your comfortable seated position.

2.   Wrap your left hand under your right armpit, holding your left scapula in place.

3.   Now slowly begin to make circles with your right arm in both directions.

4.   Stay within pain-free range as you slowly make the circles larger.

5.   Notice how large the range of movement of your shoulder joint is without the facilitation of your shoulder girdle.

6. Now repeat this on the other side noticing how the left feels compared to the right.

The following exercise focuses on isolating shoulder joint movements from thoracic spine movements.

1. Gently draw your front lower ribs back towards your spine.

2. Without moving into spinal extension slowly raise your arms up in front of you.

3. Allow your spine to move freely and raise your arms.

4. Notice how much movement took place in your spine.

5. Now you can repeat this experiment as you transition into Downward Facing Dog from being on your hands and knees.

6. Notice how much movement is coming from your shoulder joints and how much is actually coming from your spinal extension.

Thoracic mobility

All of the exercises that we discussed in Chapter 7 will also be beneficial for the shoulder girdle and shoulder joint.

Chapter 10

THE ELBOW, WRIST AND HAND

The anatomy of the elbow and forearm

The elbow joint comprises three different portions: the articulation between the ulna and humerus, that between the head of the radius and the humerus, and the articulation between the radius and ulna. All of these articulating surfaces are enveloped by a common synovial membrane, and the movements of the whole joint should be looked at together (Gray *et al.* 2005).

The portion of the joint between the ulna and humerus is a simple hinge joint and allows for movements of flexion and extension. This joint is slightly oblique, resulting in the hand being positioned away from the body when the elbow is extended but towards the midline when the elbow is flexed. The angle between the axis of the forearm and the axis of the humerus when the elbow is extended is known as the 'carrying angle'. This angle essentially prevents us from hitting our hands against our legs as we walk and swing our arms. The hand moving towards the midline when the elbow flexes allows us to easily direct the hand towards our face. In females, the average carrying angle is 13° to 16°, whereas in males, it is 11° to 14° (Morrey 2000).

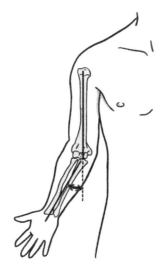

The carrying angle

In any position of flexion or extension, the radius, carrying the hand with it, can be rotated in the proximal radioulnar joint. Forward rotation of the radius so that the palm of the hand starts to turn in towards the midline and then posteriorly is called pronation. The radius essentially wraps around the ulna to form the equivalent of one strong bone that can weight-bear. Supination is the backwards rotation of the radius that results in the radius and ulna running parallel to each other and the palm of the hand facing forward. Morrey (2000) reported that the average range of supination is 75° and the average range of pronation is 70°.

The combination of the movements of flexion and extension with those of pronation and supination is essential to the accuracy of the various minute movements of the hand (Gray *et al.* 2005).

There are strong ligaments surrounding the elbow that include the anterior and posterior ligaments and the ulnar collateral and radial collateral ligaments. These act to stabilize the elbow.

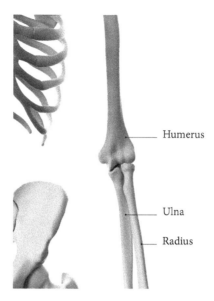

Humerus

Ulna

Radius

Anterior view of the left elbow joint

IS 'LOCKING' THE ELBOW THE SAME AS ELBOW HYPEREXTENSION?

Locking the elbow is essentially taking the joint to the end range of extension. The exact end range will be different for each person. Hyperextension of the elbow in a yoga context means extending the elbow beyond 180°, which not every student has the ability to do. The degree of extension (or hyperextension) is typically limited by the bony structure at the back of the elbow, the olecranon process of the ulna, although for some people the limiting factor will be tension in the muscle and connective tissue at the front of the elbow joint. The term hyperextension can cause confusion because hyperextension injuries of the elbow occur when the elbow is forced backwards beyond its normal range of motion. So, in a medical context, hyperextension is a pathology. Many people also assume that the ability to hyperextend the elbow joint is an indicator of systemic hypermobility. This is not necessarily the case.

Choosing to lock the elbow (which can mean hyperextension

for some people) can help to conserve energy because less muscular engagement is required to hold this position when weight-bearing. There are a few occasions when it might be best to avoid hyperextending your elbows: when doing so puts too much pressure on the wrists or shoulder joints, when this is painful for the elbow joint or when your aim is to strengthen your arm's musculature. No natural movement is intrinsically bad as long as there is awareness, control, no pain and breath.

Elbow musculature

Biceps brachii (often simply referred to as biceps) is a two-headed muscle: the long head originates from an area just above the glenoid fossa of the scapula while the short head originates from the coracoid process of the scapula. Both heads fuse and insert onto the proximal radius. Biceps flexes the elbow, is involved in flexion and abduction of the shoulder joint and is also the most powerful supinator. The long head of the biceps acts as a shoulder joint stabilizer through depression of the humeral head.

Brachialis originates from the shaft of the humerus and inserts into the proximal ulna. Brachioradialis originates from the humerus and inserts into the distal radius. Both of these muscles are involved in elbow flexion.

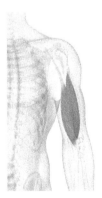

Biceps brachii

Triceps brachii (often simply referred to as triceps) is a three-headed muscle: the long head originates from an area just below the glenoid fossa of the scapula while the medial and lateral heads originate from the humerus. All heads fuse and insert into the posterior surface of the olecranon process of the ulna. Triceps is involved in elbow extension but also shoulder adduction. Triceps also helps to stabilize the shoulder joint.

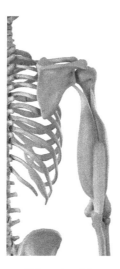

Triceps brachii

Supination is performed by biceps brachii and supinator while pronation is performed by the pronator teres and pronator quadratus.

The anatomy of the wrist

The wrist is a condyloid joint where the radius articulates with the navicular, lunate and triangular bones of the hand. The movements created in this joint are flexion, extension, abduction and adduction. When all four movements are combined, they create an elliptical movement. No rotation is possible, but the effect of rotation is obtained by the pronation and supination of the radius on the ulna.

On the anterior surface of the wrist there is the carpal tunnel through which the flexor tendons of the hand and the median nerve run. The wall of the tunnel consists of carpal bones, joint capsule, carpal ligaments and the flexor carpi radialis tendon. Carpal bones form an arch-like base for the tunnel.

Wrist musculature

Wrist flexion is defined as decreasing the angle between the palm of the hand and the forearm. It comes about by the action of flexor carpi ulnaris, flexor carpi radialis, palmaris longus and pronator teres. They all originate at the medial epicondyle of the humerus and form the common flexor tendon.

Wrist extension is defined as increasing the angle between the palm of the hand and the forearm. It is provided by extensor carpi radialis longus, extensor carpi radialis brevis and extensor carpi ulnaris. They all originate at the lateral epicondyle of the humerus.

Wrist abduction (sometimes referred to as radial deviation) is typically in the range of 15° and is produced by the flexor and extensor carpi radialis muscles.

Wrist adduction (sometimes referred to as ulnar deviation) is typically in the range of 45° and is produced by the flexor and extensor carpi ulnaris muscles.

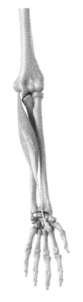 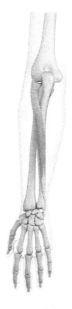

Flexor carpi radialis   Extensor carpi ulnaris

The anatomy of the hand

The hand is an extremely versatile part of our body capable of many complex and dexterous movements. Large areas of the cerebral cortex are given over to the coordination of movement and sensation in the hand. In the motor cortex the area devoted to the hands approximately equals the total area devoted to the arms, trunk and legs (Best and Taylor 1937). Similarly, the sensory areas are so large that we have the ability to recognize the shape of an object simply by holding it in our hand. The great tactile sensitivity of the hand is also largely due to the rich supply of sense organs in the hand surface itself.

The hand has a similar bony structure to the foot: the eight carpal (wrist) bones, the five metacarpals in the midsection of the hand and the phalanges in the digits. The thumb differs from the other digits in that it only has two phalanges while the others have three, and there is greater mobility in the carpometacarpal articulation. Thumb opposition refers to the ability to turn and rotate the thumb so that it can touch each fingertip of the same hand and has played a significant role in the human species being able to make tools and develop technology.

There are many extrinsic and intrinsic muscles which are involved in movement of the fingers and thumb.

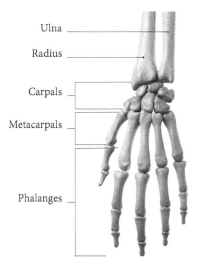

Bones of the wrist and hand

INTELLIGENT MOVEMENT PRINCIPLE – THE DIFFERENCE BETWEEN FLEXIBILITY AND MOBILITY

The terms flexibility and mobility cause quite a lot of confusion and are often used interchangeably. Their actual definitions are various depending on the source and the context. One practical way of looking at these terms that can be related directly to yoga is that mobility is about the active range of movement of a joint, i.e., the range that is under the control of the person, while flexibility is about the passive range of movement of a joint, i.e., relying on gravity and/or an external force to move into a certain range. The active range of motion is usually less than the passive range of motion.

Let's explore this topic in relation to our wrists. Place the front of your forearms together so that your wrist creases touch. Keeping your forearms touching see how wide you can separate the palms of your hands. Some of you will be able to form a 'T' shape here while most of you will probably create a 'Y' shape. Both are perfectly acceptable and demonstrate your current range of wrist extension in terms of *mobility*. Now take one hand and gently press down on the opposite palm and see how much further the wrist opens into extension. This is showing you how *flexible* your wrist joints are.

Let's now relate this to our own yoga practice. If your wrist mobility puts you in the 'Y' category then every time you place your shoulders directly above your wrists in Plank Pose (Kumbhakasana) or Tabletop Pose (Bharmanasana) you are using your body weight to move beyond your available range of wrist mobility and into the flexibility end of the spectrum. This isn't necessarily a problem for everyone, but if we are always taking our wrists into their passive range and not spending time also working on active wrist movements, we are missing a great opportunity to strengthen our wrists and keep them as healthy as possible.

Common elbow, wrist and hand injuries and conditions

In this section we will explore some of the most common elbow, wrist and hand injuries and conditions that affect our population.

Wrist pain in yoga

Wrist pain appears to be a pretty common complaint for many yoga students, particularly those who are new to the physical practice. In everyday life we use our wrists a lot for typing, texting, writing, lifting and holding objects. Most of these activities involve flexing the wrist but not extending the wrist. We also rarely bear weight on our wrists on a day-to-day basis. In yoga we do a lot of wrist extension and we tend to bear weight on our wrists quite often, and in a way that relies on wrist flexibility and not wrist mobility. In theory these factors could play a role in the incidence of wrist pain in a yoga setting.

Carpal tunnel syndrome (CTS)

CTS is believed to result from a combination of ischemia (reduced blood flow) and mechanical compression of the median nerve within the carpal tunnel of the wrist, and is a cause of pain, numbness and tingling in the upper extremities with a reduction of the grip strength and function of the affected hand. Physiological evidence indicates increased pressure within the carpal tunnel, and therefore decreased function of the median nerve at that level (Ibrahim *et al.* 2012).

It is the most common peripheral nerve entrapment syndrome worldwide (Padua *et al.* 2016) and is believed to be present in almost 4% of the general population (Atroshi *et al.* 1999). More common in females than in males, its occurrence is commonly bilaterally, with a peak age range of 40–60 years (Phalen 1966).

Most cases of CTS are labeled as idiopathic, meaning that the exact cause is unknown (Uchiyama *et al.* 2010). Neuropathic factors, such as diabetes, alcoholism, vitamin toxicity or deficiency, and exposure to toxins, can play a role in eliciting CTS symptoms. Diabetic patients have a prevalence rate of 14% and 30% without and with diabetic neuropathy, respectively (Perkins, Olaleye and Bril 2002). Extrinsic factors that can increase the volume within the tunnel include conditions that alter the fluid balance in the body. These include pregnancy, menopause, obesity, renal failure, hypothyroidism, the use of oral contraceptives and congestive heart failure (MacDermid and Doherty 2004). The prevalence of CTS during pregnancy has been reported to be around 2% (Finsen and Zeitlmann 2006).

Repetitive strain injury (RSI)

RSI can be thought of as 'overuse' injury or simply chronic injury. This is a category of injuries that result from cumulative trauma or repetitive use and stress. Overuse injuries are often the result of many repetitive minor insults. Moreover, overuse injuries occur when inadequate time is provided for the injured area of the body to heal properly. Typical examples of overuse injuries include tendinitis, bursitis, medial tibial stress syndrome and stress fractures (Yang *et al.* 2012).

Tennis elbow (lateral epicondylitis)

Tennis elbow falls under the category of RSI. It is an overuse syndrome of the common extensor tendon. Patients complain of poorly defined pain located over the lateral elbow that is typically exacerbated by activities requiring wrist extension and/or wrist supination against resistance. There will often be pain in the morning as well as after any period of time that the elbow has been held in a flexed position (Levin *et al.* 2005).

Lateral epicondylitis typically occurs in the fourth and fifth decades, with equal prevalence in women and men (Levin *et al.* 2005). A study by Shiri *et al.* (2006) reported that the prevalence of definite lateral epicondylitis was 1.3%. This study also suggested that physical load factors, smoking and obesity are strong determinants of epicondylitis. Symptoms are experienced in the dominant arm by 75% of patients (Jobe and Ciccotti 1994).

The term epicondylitis suggests an inflammatory cause; however, in all but one publication examining pathologic specimens of patients operated on for this condition, no evidence of acute or chronic inflammation is found (Boyer and Hastings 1999).

Golfer's elbow (medial epicondylitis)

Golfer's elbow is another example of RSI but is much less common than tennis elbow. It is an overuse syndrome of the common flexor tendon. Patients typically present with persistent medial-sided elbow pain that is often localized to the medial epicondyle, with radiation into the proximal forearm. Elbow pain is exacerbated by activity and is particularly bothersome during the late cocking phase in overhead throwing or during early acceleration for the thrower, tennis player or golfer (Cain *et al.* 2003).

A study by Shiri *et al.* (2006) reported that the prevalence of definite medial epicondylitis was 0.4%, although this condition may affect as many as 3.8–8.2% of patients in occupational settings (Amin, Kumar and Schickendantz 2015).

The study by Shiri *et al.* (2006) also suggested that smoking, obesity, repetitive movements and forceful activities independently of each other showed significant associations with medial epicondylitis.

Rheumatoid arthritis (RA)

RA is a chronic inflammatory, autoimmune disorder characterized by a persistent joint inflammation leading to cartilage and bone damage, disability and, eventually, to systemic complications including cardiovascular and pulmonary disorders. The most common presentation of RA is a symmetrical inflammatory polyarthritis, particularly of the hands and feet, although any synovial joint is at risk.

A study by Symmons *et al.* (2002) reported that the prevalence of RA in the UK is 1.16% in women and 0.44% in men, and that prevalence rates have decreased over the past few decades.

In a review by Picerno *et al.* (2015) the authors stated that the development of RA is attributed to a complex interaction between genetic and environmental factors and the repeated activation of innate and adaptive immune responses. These events culminate in synovial enlargement and bone destruction, leading to joint swelling and deformity, and to systemic inflammation.

In a review by McInnes and Schett (2011) the authors stated that infectious agents (including Epstein–Barr virus and E. coli) and their products have long been linked with RA, although unifying mechanisms remain elusive. The authors also reported that RA appears to be associated with periodontal disease.

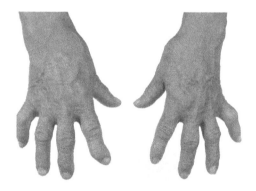

Rheumatoid arthritis in the hands

Key yoga asanas and how to adapt them

We will now explore some asanas that may present a challenge to students who are affected by the common injuries or conditions that we have discussed above and look at some of the ways that these can be adapted in order to make them more accessible.

Plank Pose (Kumbhakasana)

Plank Pose can be practiced with your forearms on the mat and elbows under the shoulders. Your knees can also be lowered; ensure you keep them behind your hips. When the hands are used as the foundation there is always the option to position the wrists slightly in front of the shoulders. Remember that not everyone can have their wrist extended to 90° without relying on external force. The hands can be placed into fists in order to keep the wrists in a more neutral position.

Downward Facing Dog (Adho Mukha Svanasana)

In the previous chapter we looked at variations of Downward Facing Dog. These included raising the height of the hands using blocks or a chair to take some load off the upper limbs. We also discussed the option of practicing this asana against a wall and Puppy Pose (Uttana Shishosana) as a useful alternative.

Students can be invited to experiment with different hand positions. Placing the hands wider than shoulder-width (to accommodate the 'carrying angle') is often a good option and the hands can also be turned out slightly. Gripping the sides of the mat by making fists can add some more support to the wrists.

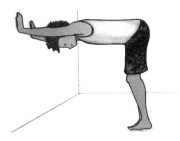

Downward Facing Dog

Tabletop Pose (Bharmanasana)

Tabletop Pose is another great example of when the option to position the wrists slightly in front of the shoulders can be used. Again, the hands can be placed into fists in order to keep the wrists in a more neutral position.

To avoid weight-bearing with the wrist a great option is to use the forearms as the front foundation, resting on bolsters or stacks of foam blocks.

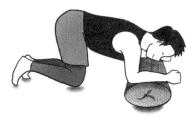

Tabletop Pose

Improving the overall health of the elbow, wrist and hand

This section addresses some effective ways in which we can all improve and maintain the health and functioning of our elbows, wrists and hands. It is intended to be a general guide for yoga practitioners and teachers and is not a replacement for the personal advice of a health professional.

Wrist mobility exercises

This is a great exercise that works specifically to develop wrist mobility.

1. Clench one fist and move your wrist in slow, controlled circles in each direction. Notice how much the bones in your forearm are also moving to facilitate the wrist movement.

2. Now repeat the exercise, this time holding on to the forearm so that the wrist joint is isolated. You can take this a stage further by isolating the wrist movements while letting go of your forearm.

3. Repeat this with your other hand.

This is a good strengthening exercise specifically for wrist extension.

1. Stand facing a wall with your hands roughly shoulder-width and shoulder-height.

2. Come to 90° of wrist extension against the wall.

3. Try to maintain this angle as you break contact with the wall.

4. This can then be practiced in a Tabletop position in order to add more load to the wrists.

5. For this variation, come to 90° of wrist extension (shoulders above your wrists) and begin to shift your shoulders back while pivoting at your wrists to maintain the 90° angle.

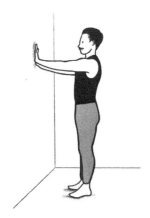

Wrist mobility exercise

Finger extension

We tend to spend a lot of time flexing our fingers throughout each day but little time extending them. Starting with your hands in a loose fist, pretend that you are flicking water at someone by rapidly and powerfully extending your fingers. You can repeat this as many times as you like.

With the palms of your hands resting on a flat surface slowly begin to lift one finger at a time. This can feel really challenging to begin with but will quickly become more manageable.

You can also wrap a resistance band around your fist and slowly extend your fingers against the resistance. There are many finger-extensor tools that you can purchase to help with this.

Supination strengthening

In yoga we tend to spend a lot of time with our forearms pronated, so it is a good idea to also focus on active supination. A simple way to add this into your practice is to turn your palms to face upwards when in Forearm Plank or Forearm Tabletop Pose. Notice if this changes the way the pose feels in the upper limbs and thoracic spine.

Co-contraction of the elbow joint

If you want to avoid moving into your end range of elbow extension, learning how to co-contract the muscles across the elbow joint is key.

1. On your hands and knees, find a gentle bend in your elbows.

2. Energetically draw your hands towards each other (without them actually moving).

3. Hold this for a few breaths and notice if it is more challenging to straighten your arms.

4. Release this action and rest for a moment.

5. To make this action more challenging you can lift your knees a couple of inches off the floor and repeat the same exercise.

6. You can also try to repeat this action while in Downward Facing Dog (Adho Mukha Svanasana).

Shoulder girdle and shoulder joint mobility

All of the exercises that we discussed in the previous chapter will also play a role in improving the health of your elbows, wrists and hands.

Part 4

COMMON
MEDICAL
CONDITIONS

A free online class focusing on managing stress
can be found at https://lddy.no/pat9.

Cardiovascular disease (CVD)

CVD is the leading cause of death for both men and women of most racial and ethnic groups in the United States (Heron 2019).

Coronary artery disease (CAD) is the most common type of CVD in the US. It is sometimes called coronary heart disease or ischemic heart disease. CAD is caused by plaque buildup in the wall of the arteries that supply blood to the heart (called coronary arteries). Plaque is made up of cholesterol deposits, and buildup of this causes the inside of the arteries to narrow over time, which can partially or totally block the blood flow. This process is called atherosclerosis.

High blood pressure, high cholesterol and smoking are all risk factors that could lead to CVD and stroke. In 2009–2010, approximately 46.5% of US adults aged 20 and over had at least one of these three risk factors (Fryar, Chen and Li 2012). Several other medical conditions and lifestyle choices can also put people at a higher risk for heart disease, including diabetes, obesity, unhealthy diet, physical inactivity and excessive alcohol use.

Blood pressure is the pressure that is exerted on the artery wall as blood is ejected from the heart. This pressure is essential for blood to travel throughout the body. High blood pressure (HBP or hypertension) is when blood pressure is consistently too high. The primary way that HBP causes harm is by increasing the workload of the heart and blood vessels, making them work harder and less efficiently. Over time, the force and friction of HBP damages the delicate tissues inside the arteries. In turn, cholesterol forms plaque along tiny tears in the artery walls, signifying the start of atherosclerosis.

As with all of the conditions and injuries that we have discussed throughout this handbook it is important that the student has been given the go-ahead by their healthcare practitioner before practicing yoga.

Students with controlled HBP can typically practice in the same way that someone with normal blood pressure would. Students with uncontrolled HBP need to be particularly mindful when it comes to inversions because elevating the heart above the head and the torso and legs above the heart will raise the blood pressure. A partially inverted posture like Downward Facing Dog (Adho Mukha Svanasana), where the heart is only slightly above the head and the legs are not elevated, may only slightly increase the blood pressure. Any of the modifications for Downward Facing Dog that we have explored throughout the handbook can be adopted, particularly if the student feels too much pressure in their head or feels short of breath. Supported Bridge Pose (Setu Bandha Sarvangasana), lying on bolsters with the legs horizontal and feet at hip level, increases pressure in the head a little more. Students should always be given the option to come out of the asana if they feel uncomfortable in any way. Shoulderstand (Salamba Sarvangasana) and Headstand (Sirsasana) should be avoided when a student has uncontrolled HBP.

A meta-analysis by Cramer *et al.* (2014a) revealed evidence for clinically important effects of yoga on most biological CVD risk factors. The authors state that yoga can be considered as a supporting intervention for the general population and for patients with increased risk of CVD. A systematic review and meta-analysis by Hagins *et al.* (2013) reported that yoga can be preliminarily recommended as an effective intervention for reducing blood pressure.

Diabetes mellitus

Diabetes is a chronic, metabolic disease characterized by elevated levels of blood glucose (hyperglycemia), which leads over time to serious damage to the heart, blood vessels, eyes, kidneys and nerves. Type 1 diabetes, once known as juvenile diabetes or insulin-dependent diabetes, is a chronic condition in which the pancreas produces little or no insulin by itself. More common than this is type 2 diabetes, which usually presents in adults and occurs when the body becomes resistant to insulin or does not make enough insulin. In the past three decades the prevalence of type 2 diabetes has risen dramatically in countries of all income levels (Shaw, Sicree and Zimmet 2010). Gestational diabetes is hyperglycemia with blood glucose values above normal but below that diagnostic of diabetes, occurring during pregnancy. Women with gestational diabetes are at an increased risk of complications during pregnancy and at delivery. They and their children are also at increased risk of type 2 diabetes in the future. In 2014, 8.5% of US adults aged 18 years and older had type 2 diabetes (Xu *et al.* 2018).

If a student has diabetes it is always a good idea to find out how they are doing today and if exercise tends to affect their glucose levels significantly. You might want to ask if they have tested their blood glucose level before they arrived for class. If a student has very high or low blood sugar levels, exercise could aggravate their condition. If a student has a hypoglycemic episode (low blood glucose) during the practice they might become irrational, moody or even appear like they are drunk. They will need to rest and have a snack.

In Chapter 1 we briefly explored diabetic neuropathy. Diabetic neuropathy (nerve damage) is the most common complication associated with diabetes (Singh *et al.* 2014) with at least half of all diabetic patients developing some form of neuropathy during their lifetime. Diabetic neuropathy is primarily a disorder of sensory nerves. Sensory symptoms such as pain, tingling, prickling sensations and numbness start in the toes and over time affect the upper limbs in a distribution classically described as a 'stocking and glove' pattern. Only much later in the course of the disease is there evidence of motor nerve dysfunction, with distal weakness of the toes and, in extreme cases, the ankles and calves. Diabetic neuropathy can lead to foot ulceration and amputation, gait disturbance, fall-related injury and neuropathic pain. For students who have had diabetes for some time it is important to talk about their risk of falling and adapt standing poses accordingly.

A meta-analysis by Cui *et al.* (2017) suggested that yoga can benefit adult patients with type 2 diabetes mellitus.

Asthma

Asthma is a chronic lung disease caused by the contraction of smooth muscle surrounding the airways, making it difficult to breathe and resulting in coughing and wheezing. It is estimated that 5% of adults worldwide have bronchial asthma (Sathyaprabha, Murthy and Murthy 2001).

Students with asthma need to be encouraged to rest if they feel uncomfortable or short of breath during the practice (the same goes for all students). I would strongly recommend taking a dedicated pranayama teacher training course before teaching pranayama in a one-to-one or group setting.

Although anecdotally yoga can be very beneficial for many students who have asthma, currently there is a lack of quality studies that look at yoga as a therapeutic intervention for asthma. A systematic review and meta-analysis by Cramer *et al.* (2014b) reported that yoga cannot be considered a routine intervention for asthmatic patients at this point. It can be considered a supporting intervention or an alternative to breathing exercises for asthma patients interested in complementary interventions. A systematic review by Posadzki and Ernst (2011) stated that the belief that yoga alleviates asthma is not supported by sound evidence and more rigorous trials are warranted.

Pregnancy

As a general rule, women who have a regular yoga practice prior to their pregnancy can continue as usual during the first trimester. As always, it is good to establish that the student has been given the go-ahead by their healthcare practitioner. Modifications will generally be required during the second and third trimester. Each pregnancy is unique, and it is up to the expectant mother to decide what is best for her during this time. As a teacher you must communicate clearly and stick to your own personal boundaries around teaching pregnant women. Many women decide to commence yoga for the first time once pregnant. In this case participation should ideally be in specifically designed pre-natal classes by a qualified teacher. Specialist pre- and post-natal training is essential if you wish to work with pregnant women. Particular cautions when teaching students who are pregnant include: overexertion and overheating, overstretching (due to the hormone relaxin), undue pressure on the uterus during twisting postures, jarring the uterus during transitions, balance postures due to the change in center of gravity, lying flat and inversions (due to the change in center of gravity and already rising blood pressure).

Osteoporosis

Osteoporosis is a systemic skeletal condition characterized by low bone mass and microarchitectural deterioration of bone tissue that increases bone fragility and risk for fractures (US DoHHS 2004). Osteoporosis may occur without a known cause, or secondary to another condition including corticosteroid therapy, excessive alcohol use, low calcium intake, vitamin D deficiency, smoking, antiepileptic drug use, thyrotoxicosis, primary hyperparathyroidism, chronic liver or kidney disease, rheumatoid arthritis and diabetes.

Osteoporosis is diagnosed in individuals on the basis of the presence of a fragility fracture or by bone mass measurement criteria. A fragility fracture results from forces that would not normally cause a fracture, such as a hip or wrist fracture from falling from standing height or a vertebral compression fracture. Although specific fracture sites have been considered more characteristic of osteoporosis, fractures occurring at nearly every anatomical site have been associated with osteoporosis. It is estimated that 30–50% of women and 15–30% of men will have an osteoporotic fracture in their lifetime (US DoHHS 2004).

When teaching a student who has osteoporosis it is important to adapt standing poses in order to decrease the risk of the student falling. It is also worth noting that while people who have osteoporosis will benefit from gentle spinal movement, there needs to be a degree of caution here, due to the increased risk of vertebral fracture. Spinal flexion, extension, rotation and lateral flexion should all be practiced in a particularly mindful, gentle and controlled way while limiting the range of movement. Rolling up from a standing forward fold can put a significant amount of stress on each level of the spine during the transition, so a good option here is to place the hands at the back of the legs to reduce the load or to rise up with a more neutral spine and the hands on the hips.

A systematic review by McCaffrey and Park (2012) looked at the benefits of yoga for musculoskeletal disorders including osteoporosis. Noting that they were only able to include three studies on osteoporosis in their review due to their inclusion criteria, they reported that yoga has a positive impact on osteoporosis. A ten-year study by Lu *et al.* (2016) suggested that yoga can reverse bone loss that has reached the stages of osteoporosis.

Hypermobility

Joint hypermobility is a term used to describe the capability of joints to move beyond normal limits. It can exist by itself or be a part of a more complex diagnosis. Those with joint hypermobility in a couple of joints (fewer than five) can be described as having localized joint hypermobility. Those with joint hypermobility in five or more joints can be described as having generalized joint hypermobility. Joint hypermobility can be symptomless apart from the unusual mobility, but there is a series of other symptoms that result from that mobility including microtrauma (dislocation, subluxations and connected soft tissue damage), persistent pain and disturbed proprioception.

Hypermobility spectrum disorders are a group of conditions related to joint hypermobility. Hypermobility spectrum disorders are intended to be diagnosed after other possible answers are excluded, such as any of the Ehlers-Danlos syndromes.

The Ehlers-Danlos syndromes are a group of connective tissue disorders that can be inherited and are varied both in how they affect the body and in their genetic causes. They are generally characterized by joint hypermobility (joints that stretch further than normal), skin hyperextensibility (skin that can be stretched further than normal) and tissue fragility. The Ehlers-Danlos syndromes are currently classified into 13 subtypes according to the signs and symptoms that are manifested.

Teaching yoga to a student who is hypermobile is a big topic and I am going to distill this into a few key principles. This information is by no means exhaustive and it is also good to know that these principles tend to be good practice for working with all students. Moving away from the common belief that yoga is all about flexibility and educating students on the internal focus of the yoga practice is really important. Focusing on the quality and control of the movements that are being made rather than on a goal of end range of movement will be helpful. This comes back to the principle of mobility versus flexibility that we explored early in the handbook. Encouraging students to micro-bend their elbows and knees, hug their muscles to their bones and draw their arm bones and thigh bones into the sockets can all be useful cues to develop stability and a sense of containment. As always, try to avoid using fear-based language. Balance and stability can be a particular challenge for students who are hypermobile. All of the options that we have explored throughout the handbook in terms of making balance poses accessible should be helpful here. When an asana is being held for some time always offer the option for students to move out of the asana at any time. It is also important to note that students who are hypermobile will still experience tightness, so stretching can be really important. Having compassion is absolutely crucial: working with proprioception and mobility can be a long journey and both physically and mentally exhausting for hypermobile people.

Depression and anxiety

This is another huge topic and tackling it in any real depth goes beyond the scope of this handbook, but I do want to briefly touch on this important subject. Having an understanding of and compassion for mental health conditions is an important part of teaching yoga. However, this does not mean that we take on the role of a trained therapist. When enquiring about your students' wellbeing try to use language that is inclusive of mental health issues. Being a good listener is often the most helpful and the most appropriate thing for a teacher to focus on. If you have experienced working with a therapist, you might find that you are open to sharing their details with a student if that feels appropriate. Be open to challenging your pre-existing beliefs about what a specific asana should look like. A good example of this is Corpse Pose (Savasana). Lying on one's back with eyes closed might not feel like a comfortable option for someone who has anxiety. Lying on one's side in a fetal position, or a prone position, might feel like a much more accessible choice. If options are not offered, then it is much less likely that a student will adopt a position that actually works for them.

Depression

Depression is an extremely common illness worldwide, with more than 264 million people affected (GBD 2017 Disease and Injury Incidence and Prevalence Collaborators 2018). The World Health Organization (2012) projects that depression will be the world's leading disease by 2030.

A systematic review and meta-analysis by Cramer *et al.* (2013b) concluded that yoga could be considered a supplementary treatment option for patients with depressive disorders and individuals with elevated levels of depression.

Anxiety

An estimated 31.1% of US adults experience an anxiety disorder at some time in their lives and an estimated 19.1% of US adults had an anxiety disorder in the past year (Harvard Medical School 2007).

In a systematic review by Sharma and Haider (2013b) looking at the effect that yoga has on anxiety, a total of 27 studies met their inclusion criteria and, of these, 19 studies demonstrated a significant reduction in anxiety. In a systematic review by Pascoe and Bauer (2015) the 25 randomized control studies that were included provided preliminary evidence to suggest that yoga practice leads to better regulation of the sympathetic nervous system, as well as a decrease in depressive and anxious symptoms in a range of populations.

GLOSSARY OF ANATOMICAL TERMS

Abduction: movement of a limb away from the midline in a vertical plane.

Adduction: movement of a limb towards the midline in a vertical plane.

Anatomical position: the erect position of the body with the face directed forward, the arms at the side and the palms of the hands facing forward, used as a reference in describing the relation of body parts to one another.

Anterior: closer to the front of the body.

Bursa: a closed, fluid-filled sac that functions as a gliding surface to reduce friction between tissues of the body.

Deep: further from the surface of the body.

Distal: further from the torso, when referring to a part of the limbs.

Extension: movement that increases the angle between two body parts.

Flexion: movement that decreases the angle between two body parts.

Foramen: an opening or passage in a bone.

Frontal plane: a vertical plane that separates the body into front and back portions. This is sometimes referred to as the coronal plane. (Refer to the figure below.)

Horizontal abduction: movement of a limb away from the midline in a horizontal plane.

Horizontal adduction: movement of a limb towards the midline in a horizontal plane.

Inferior: further away from the head, when referring to part of the torso.

Lateral: further from the midline of the body.

Medial: closer to the midline of the body.

Posterior: closer to the back of the body.

Proximal: closer to the torso, when referring to a part of the limbs.

Rotation: a twisting movement that can occur within the spine or at a ball-and-socket joint. For a ball-and-socket joint the movement that brings the front surface of the limb toward the midline of the body is called internal (or medial) rotation. Conversely, rotation of the limb so that the front surface moves away from the midline is external (or lateral) rotation.

Sagittal plane: a vertical plane that separates the body into right and left sections. (Refer to the figure below.)

Superficial: closer to the surface of the body.

Superior: closer to the head, when referring to part of the torso.

Transverse plane: a horizontal plane that separates the body into upper and lower sections. (Refer to the figure below.)

Valgus: displacement of part of a limb away from the midline of the body.

Varus: displacement of part of a limb towards the midline of the body.

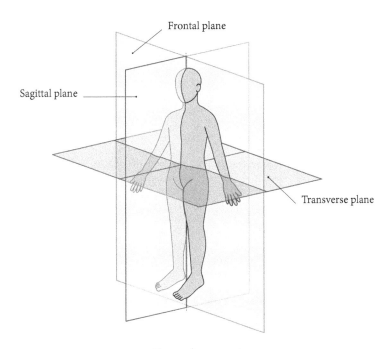

Planes of movement

REFERENCES

Ailon, T., Shaffrey, C., Lenke, L., Harrop, J. and Smith, J. (2015) 'Progressive spinal kyphosis in the aging population.' *Neurosurgery 77*, suppl 1, S164–S172.

Allen, R. and Gross, M. (2003) 'Toe flexors strength and passive extension range of motion of the first metatarsophalangeal joint in individuals with plantar fasciopathy.' *J Orthop Sports Phys Ther 33*, 8, 468–478.

Aman, J., Elangovan, N., Yeh, I. and Konczak, J. (2015) 'The effectiveness of proprioceptive training for improving motor function: A systematic review.' *Frontiers in Human Neuroscience 8*, 1075.

Amin, N., Kumar, N. and Schickendantz, M. (2015) 'Medial epicondylitis: Evaluation and management.' *J American Academy of Orthopaedic Surgeons 23*, 6, 348–355.

An, J., Jeon, D., Jung, W., Yang, I., Lim, W. and Ahn, S. (2015) 'Influence of temporomandibular joint disc displacement on craniocervical posture and hyoid bone position.' *Am J Orthod Dentofacial Orthop 147*, 1, 72–79.

Anandacoomarasamy, A. and Barnsley, L. (2005) 'Long term outcomes of inversion ankle injuries.' *Br J Sports Med 39*, 1–4.

Anderson, J. and Felson, D. (1988) 'Factors associated with osteoarthritis of the knee in the first national Health and Nutrition Examination Survey (HANES I): Evidence for an association with overweight, race, and physical demands of work.' *Am J Epidemiol 128*, 179–189.

Anderson, J. and Trinkaus, E. (1998) 'Patterns of sexual, bilateral and interpopulational variation in human femoral neck-shaft angles.' *J Anat 192*, 279–285.

Andersson, E., Oddsson, L., Grundström, H. and Thorstensson, A. (1995) 'The role of the psoas and iliacus muscles for stability and movement of the lumbar spine, pelvis and hip.' *Scand J Med Sci Sports 5*, 1, 10–16.

Andersson, G. (1997) 'The Epidemiology of Spinal Disorders.' In J. Frymoyer (ed.) *The Adult Spine: Principles and Practice, 2nd ed.* New York: Raven Press.

Andrianakos, A., Kontelis, L., Karamitsos, D., Aslanidis, S. *et al.* (2006) 'Prevalence of symptomatic knee, hand and hip osteoarthritis in Greece: The ESORDIG study.' *J Rheumatology 33*, 2507–2513.

Arnoczky, S. and Warren, R. (1982) 'Microvasculature of the human meniscus.' *Am J Sports Med 10*, 2, 90–95.

Askling, C., Lund, H., Saartok, T. and Thorstensson, A. (2002) 'Self-reported hamstring injuries in student-dancers.' *Scand J Med Sci Sports 12*, 230–235.

Atroshi, I., Gummesson, C., Johnsson, R., Ornstein, E., Ranstam, J. and Rosen, I. (1999) 'Prevalence of carpal tunnel syndrome in a general population.' *JAMA 282*, 2, 153–158.

Bakker, E., Verhagen, A., van Trijffel, E., Lucas, C. and Koes, B. (2009) 'Spinal mechanical load as a risk factor for low back pain: A systematic review of prospective cohort studies.' *Spine 34*, 8, 281–293.

Balduini, F. and Tetzlaff, J. (1982) 'Historical perspectives on injuries of the ligaments of the ankle.' *Clin Sports Med 1*, 3–12.

Ballmer, P. and Jakob, R. (1988) 'The non-operative treatment of isolated complete tears of the medial collateral ligament of the knee: A prospective study.' *Arch Orthop Trauma Surg 107*, 273–276.

Bandholm, T., Boysen, L., Haugaard, S., Kreutzfeldt Zebis, M. and Bencke, J. (2008) 'The foot medial longitudinal-arch deformation during quiet standing and gait in subjects with medial tibial stress syndrome.' *J Foot Ankle Surg 47*, 2, 89–95.

Bartolozzi, A., Andreychik, D. and Ahmad, S. (1994) 'Determinants of outcome in the treatment of rotator cuff disease.' *Clin Orthop Relat Res 308*, 90–97.

Basmajian, J. and Stecko, G. (1963) 'The role of muscles in arch support of the foot.' *J Bone Joint Surg Am 45*, 1184–1190.

Bates, S. and Ginsberg, J. (2001) 'Pregnancy and deep vein thrombosis.' *Semin Vasc Med 1*, 1, 97–104.

Beaton, L. and Anson, B. (1938) 'The sciatic nerve and the piriformis muscle: Their interrelation and possible cause of coccygodynia.' *J Bone Joint Surg Am 20*, 686–688.

Beattie, P. (2008) 'Current understanding of lumbar intervertebral disc degeneration: A review with emphasis upon etiology, pathophysiology, and lumbar magnetic resonance imaging findings.' *J Orthop Sports Phys Ther 38*, 6, 329–340.

Becker, I., Woodley, S. and Stringer, M. (2010) 'The adult human pubic symphysis: a systematic review.' *J Anat 217*, 475–487.

Been, E. and Kalichman, L. (2014) 'Lumbar lordosis.' *Spine J 14*, 1, 87–97.

Benjamin, D., van de Water, A. and Peiris, C. (2014) 'Effects of exercise on diastasis of the rectus abdominis muscle in the antenatal and postnatal periods: A systematic review.' *Physiotherapy 100*, 1, 1–8.

Benvenuti, F., Ferrucci, L., Guralnik, J., Gangemi, S. and Baroni, A. (1995) 'Foot pain and disability in older persons: An epidemiologic survey.' *J Am Geriatr Soc 43*, 479–484.

Benyamin, R., Singh, V., Parr, A., Conn, A., Diwan, S. and Abdi, S. (2009) 'Systematic review of the effectiveness of cervical epidurals in the management of chronic neck pain.' *Pain Physician 12*, 1, 137–157.

Berger, R. and Doyle, S. (2019) 'Spondylolysis 2019 update.' *Curr Opin Pediatr 31*, 1, 61–68.

Bess, S., Boachie-Adjei, O., Burton, D., Cunningham, M. *et al.* (2009) 'Pain and disability determine treatment modality for older patients with adult scoliosis, while deformity guides treatment for younger patients.' *Spine 34*, 20, 2186–2190.

Best, C. and Taylor, N. (1937) *Physiological Basis of Medical Practice.* Baltimore, MD: Williams and Wilkins.

Bhoir, M. (2014) 'Prevalence of flat foot among 18–25 years old physiotherapy students: Cross sectional study.' *Indian J Basic Applied Med Research 3*, 4, 272–278.

Bialosky, J., Bishop, M. and Cleland, J. (2010) 'Individual expectation: An overlooked, but pertinent, factor in the treatment of individuals experiencing musculoskeletal pain.' *Phys Ther 90*, 9, 1345–1355.

Biggs, E., Meulders, A. and Vlaeyen, J. (2016) 'The Neuroscience of Pain and Fear.' In M. al'Absi and M. Arve Flaten (eds) *Neuroscience of Pain, Stress, and Emotion.* Cambridge, MA: Academic Press.

Bø, K. (2004) 'Pelvic floor muscle training is effective in treatment of female stress urinary incontinence, but how does it work?' *Int Urogynecol J 15*, 76–84.

Bø, K. (2012) 'Pelvic floor muscle training in treatment of female stress urinary incontinence, pelvic organ prolapse and sexual dysfunction.' *World Journal of Urology 30*, 437–443.

Boden, S., McCowin, P., Davis, D., Dina, T., Mark, A. and Wiesel, S. (1990) 'Abnormal magnetic-resonance scans of the cervical spine in asymptomatic subjects: A prospective investigation.' *J Bone Joint Surg Am 72*, 1178–1184.

Bogduk, N. and Mercer, S. (2000) 'Biomechanics of the cervical spine. I: Normal kinematics.' *Clin Biomech 15*, 633–648.

Boruta, P., Bishop, J., Grant Braly, W. and Tullos, H. (1990) 'Acute ankle ligament injuries; a literature review.' *Foot Ankle 11*, 107–113.

Botsford, D., Esses, S. and Ogilvie-Harris, D. (1994) 'In vivo diurnal variation in intervertebral disc volume and morphology.' *Spine 19*, 8, 935–940.

Boyer, M. and Hastings, H. (1999) 'Lateral tennis elbow: "Is there any science out there?"' *Journal of Shoulder and Elbow Surgery 8*, 5, 481–491.

Boyle-Walker, K., Gabard, D., Bietsch, E., Masek-VanArsdale, D. and Robinson, B. (1997) 'A profile of patients with adhesive capsulitis.' *J Hand Ther 10*, 222–228.

Bozkurt, M., Yumru, A. and Şahin, L. (2014) 'Pelvic floor dysfunction, and effects of pregnancy and mode of delivery on pelvic floor.' *Taiwanese Journal of Obstetrics and Gynecology 53*, 4, 452–458.

Bråten, M., Terjesen, T. and Rossvoll, I. (1992) 'Femoral anteversion in normal adults.' *Acta Orthop Scand 63*, 1, 29–32.

Brattström, H. (1964) 'Shape of the intercondylar groove normally and in recurrent dislocation of the patella.' *Acta Orthop Scand 68*, 1–44.

Brewin, J., Hill, M. and Ellis, H. (2009) 'The prevalence of cervical ribs in a London population.' *Clin Anat 22*, 331–336.

Briggs, A., Greig, A., Wark, J., Fazzalari, N. and Bennell, K. (2004) 'A review of anatomical and mechanical factors affecting vertebral body integrity.' *International Journal of Medical Sciences 1*, 3, 170–180.

Brinjikji, W., Luetmer, P., Comstock, B., Bresnahan, B. *et al.* (2015) 'Systematic literature review of imaging features of spinal degeneration in asymptomatic populations.' *American Journal of Neuroradiology 36*, 4, 811–816.

Buchholtz, K., Lambert, M., Bosch, A. and Burgess, T. (2018) 'Calf muscle architecture and function in ultra runners and low physical activity individuals: A comparative review.' *Transl Sports Med 1*, 250–256.

Bueno, A., Pilgaard, M., Hulme, A., Forsberg, P. *et al.* (2018) 'Injury prevalence across sports: A descriptive analysis on a representative sample of the Danish population.' *Injury Epidemiology 5*, 1, 6.

Cain, E., Dugas, J., Wolf, R. and Andrews, J. (2003) 'Elbow injuries in throwing athletes: A current concepts review.' *Am J Sports Med 31*, 4, 621–635.

Carreiro, J. (2009) *Pediatric Manual Medicine*. London: Churchill Livingstone.

Carroll, L., Hogg-Johnson, S., van der Velde, G., Haldeman, S. and Holm, L. (2008) 'Course and prognostic factors for neck pain in the general population.' *Eur Spine J 17*, suppl 1, S75–S82.

Centers for Disease Control and Prevention (CDC) (2001) 'Prevalence of disabilities and associated health conditions among adults–United States, 1999.' *JAMA 285*, 12, 1571–1572.

Chang, R., Kent-Braun, J. and Hamill, J. (2012) 'Use of MRI for volume estimation of tibialis posterior and plantar intrinsic foot muscles in healthy and chronic plantar fasciopathy limbs.' *Clinical Biomechanics 27*, 5, 500–505.

Cheatham, S., Kolber, M., Cain, M. and Lee, M. (2015) 'The effects of self-myofascial release using a foam roll or roller massager on joint range of motion, muscle recovery and performance: A systematic review.' *Int J Sports Phys Ther 10*, 6, 827–838.

Chen, T., Rozen, W., Pan, W., Ashton, M., Richardson, M. and Taylor, G. (2009) 'The arterial anatomy of the Achilles tendon: Anatomical study and clinical implications.' *Clin Anat 22*, 377–385.

Chiu, C., Chuang, T., Chang, K., Wu, C., Lin, P. and Hsu, W. (2015) 'The probability of spontaneous regression of lumbar herniated disc: A systematic review.' *Clin Rehabil 29*, 2, 184–195.

Cilli, F. and Akçaoğlu, M. (2005) 'The incidence of accessory bones of the foot and their clinical significance.' *Acta Orthop Traumatol Turc 39*, 3, 243–246.

Ciol, M., Deyo, R., Howell, E. and Kreif, S. (1996) 'An assessment of surgery for spinal stenosis: Time trends, geographic variations, complications, and reoperations.' *J Am Geriatr Soc 44*, 285–290.

Codman, E. (1934) *The Shoulder*. Boston, MA: Thomas Todd Co.

Cohen, S. (2015) 'Epidemiology, diagnosis, and treatment of neck pain.' *Mayo Clin Proc 90*, 2, 284–299.

Côté, P., van der Velde, G., Cassidy, J., Hogg-Johnson, S. *et al.* (2009) 'The burden and determinants of neck pain in workers: Results of the Bone and Joint Decade 2000–2010 Task Force on Neck Pain and Its Associated Disorders.' *J Manipulative Physiol Ther 32*, 2, S70–S86.

Cramer, H., Lauche, R., Haller, H. and Dobos, G. (2013a) 'A systematic review and meta-analysis of yoga for low back pain.' *The Clinical Journal of Pain 29*, 5, 450–460.

Cramer, H., Lauche, R., Langhorst, J. and Dobos, G. (2013b) 'Yoga for depression: A systematic review and meta-analysis.' *Depression Anxiety 30*, 1068–1083.

Cramer, H., Lauche, R., Haller, H., Steckhan, N., Michalsen, A. and Dobos, G. (2014a) 'Effects of yoga on cardiovascular disease risk factors: A systematic review and meta-analysis.' *International Journal of Cardiology 173*, 2, 170–183.

Cramer, H., Posadzki, P., Dobos, G. and Langhorst, J. (2014b) 'Yoga for asthma: A systematic review and meta-analysis.' *Annals of Allergy, Asthma & Immunology 112*, 6, 503–510.

Cramer, H., Quinker, D., Schumann, D., Wardle, J., Dobos, G. and Lauche, R. (2019) 'Adverse effects of yoga: A national cross-sectional survey.' *BMC Complement Altern Med 19*, 1, 190.

Cramer, H., Ward, L., Saper, R., Fishbein, D., Dobos, G. and Lauche, R. (2015) 'The safety of yoga: A systematic review and meta-analysis of randomized controlled trials.' *American Journal of Epidemiology 182*, 4, 281–293.

Croft, P., Coggon, D., Cruddas, M. and Cooper, C. (1992) 'Osteoarthritis of the hip: An occupational disease in farmers.' *BMJ 304*, 1269–1272.

Cross, M., Smith, E., Hoy, D., Nolte, S. *et al.* (2014) 'The global burden of hip and knee osteoarthritis: Estimates from the global burden of disease 2010 study.' *Ann Rheum Dis 73*, 1323–1330.

Cui, J., Yan, J., Yan, L., Pan, L., Le, J. and Guo, Y. (2017) 'Effects of yoga in adults with type 2 diabetes mellitus: A meta-analysis.' *J Diabetes Investig 8*, 201–209.

Dagenais, S., Garbedian, S. and Wai, E. (2009) 'Systematic review of the prevalence of radiographic primary hip osteoarthritis.' *Clinical Orthopaedics and Related Research 467*, 3, 623–637.

Daghighi, M., Pouriesa, M., Maleki, M., Fouladi, D. *et al.* (2014) 'Migration patterns of herniated disc fragments: A study on 1,020 patients with extruded lumbar disc herniation.' *Spine J 14*, 1970–1977.

Damasceno, G., Ferreira, A., Nogueira, L., Reis, F., Andrade, I. and Meziat-Filho, N. (2018) 'Text neck and neck pain in 18 to 21-year-old young adults.' *European Spine Journal 27*, 1249–1254.

Dankaerts, W., O'Sullivan, P., Burnett, A. and Straker, L. (2009) 'Discriminating healthy controls and two clinical subgroups of nonspecific chronic low back pain patients using trunk muscle activation and lumbosacral kinematics of postures and movements: A statistical classification model.' *Spine 34*, 1610–1618.

Devereaux, M. (2009) 'Low back pain.' *Medical Clinics of North America 93*, 2, 477–501.

Deyo, R. (2002) 'Diagnostic evaluation of LBP: Reaching a specific diagnosis is often impossible.' *Archives of Internal Medicine 162*, 1444–1447.

Dixit, R. (2017) 'Low Back Pain.' In G. Firestein, R. Budd, S. Gabriel, I. McInnes and J. O'Dell (eds) *Kelley and Firestein's Textbook of Rheumatology, 10th ed.* Amsterdam: Elsevier.

Donley, E. and Loyd, J. (2019) *Anatomy, Thorax, Wall Movements.* Treasure Island, FL: StatPearls Publishing. Accessed on 17/06/2020 at www.ncbi.nlm.nih.gov/books/NBK526023.

Dreyfuss, P., Cole, A. and Pauza, K. (1995) 'Sacroiliac joint injection techniques.' *Phys Med Rehabil Clin North Am 6*, 785–813.

Dreyfuss, P., Dreyer, S., Cole, A. and Mayo, K. (2004) 'Sacroiliac joint pain.' *J Am Acad Orthop Surg 12*, 255–265.

Drosos, G. and Pozo, J. (2004) 'The causes and mechanisms of meniscal injuries in the sporting and non-sporting environment in an unselected population.' *Knee 11*, 143–149.

Dubois, B. and Esculier, J.-F. (2019) 'Soft tissue injuries simply need PEACE & LOVE.' *British Journal of Sports Medicine Blog.* Accessed on 17/06/2020 at https://blogs.bmj.com/bjsm/2019/04/26/soft-tissue-injuries-simply-need-peace-love.

Egund, N., Olsson, T., Schmid, H. and Selvik, G. (1978) 'Movements in the sacroiliac joints demonstrated with roentgen stereophotogrammetric analysis.' *Acta Radiol Diagn 19*, 833–845.

Ellison, A. and Berg, E. (1985) 'Embryology, anatomy, and function of the anterior cruciate ligament.' *Orthop Clin N Am 16*, 3–14.

Emami, M., Ghahramani, M., Abdinejad, F. and Namazi, H. (2007) 'Q-angle: An invaluable parameter for evaluation of anterior knee pain.' *Archives of Iranian Medicine 10*, 1, 24–26.

Englund, M., Felson, T., Guermazi, A., Roemer, F. *et al.* (2011) 'Risk factors for medial meniscal pathology on knee MRI in older US adults: A multicentre prospective cohort study.' *Ann Rheum Dis 70*, 1733–1739.

Englund, M., Guermazi, A. and Lohmander, S. (2009) 'The role of the meniscus in knee osteoarthritis: A cause or consequence?' *Radiologic Clinics 47*, 4, 703–712.

Esses, S. and Botsford, D. (1997) 'Surgical Anatomy and Operative Approaches to the Sacrum.' In J. Frymoyer (ed.) *The Adult Spine: Principles and Practice, 2nd ed.* Philadelphia, PA: Lippincott-Raven.

Evans, C., Fowkes, F., Ruckley, C. and Lee, A. (1999) 'Prevalence of varicose veins and chronic venous insufficiency in men and women in the general population: Edinburgh Vein Study.' *J Epidemiol Comm Health 53*, 149–153.

Fanelli, G. and Harris, J. (2006) 'Surgical treatment of acute medial collateral ligament and posteromedial corner injuries of the knee.' *Sports Med Arthrosc Rev 14*, 78–83.

Fardon, D., Williams, A., Dohring, E., Murtagh, F., Gabriel Rothman, S. and Sze, G. (2014) 'Lumbar disc nomenclature: Version 2.0. Recommendations of the combined task forces of the North American Spine Society, the American Society of Spine Radiology and the American Society of Neuroradiology.' *Spine J 14*, 11, 2525–2545.

Farias, M., Oliveira, B., Rocha, T. and Caiaffo, V. (2012) 'Morphological and morphometric analysis of psoas minor muscle in cadavers.' *J Morphol Sci 29*, 4, 202–205.

Fathallah, F., Marras, W. and Wright, P. (1995) 'Diurnal variation in trunk kinematics during a typical work shift.' *J Spinal Disord 8*, 1, 20–25.

Fayad, F., Lefevre-Colau, M., Poiraudeau, S. and Fermanian, J. (2004) 'Chronicity, recurrence, and return to work in low back pain: Common prognostic factors.' *Ann Readapt Med Phys 47*, 179–189.

Felson, T., Niu, J., Gross, D., Englund, M. *et al.* (2013) 'Valgus malalignment is a risk factor for lateral knee osteoarthritis incidence and progression: Findings from the multicenter osteoarthritis study and the osteoarthritis initiative.' *Arthritis & Rheumatism 65*, 355–362.

Ferguson, S., Bryant, J., Ganz, R. and Ito, K. (2003) 'An in vitro investigation of the acetabular labral seal in hip joint mechanics.' *Journal of Biomechanics 36*, 171–178.

Finsen, V. and Zeitlmann, H. (2006) 'Carpal tunnel syndrome during pregnancy.' *Scand J Plast Reconstr Surg Hand Surg 40*, 1, 41–45.

Fischer, B. and Mitteroecker, P. (2017) 'Allometry and sexual dimorphism in the human pelvis.' *The Anatomical Record 300*, 698–705.

Fitzgerald, J. and Newman, P. (1976) 'Degenerative spondylolisthesis.' *J Bone Joint Surg Br 58*, 184–192.

Flandry, F. and Hommel, G. (2011) 'Normal anatomy and biomechanics of the knee.' *Sports Medicine and Arthroscopy Review 19*, 2, 82–92.

Fon, G., Pitt, M. and Thies, A. (1980) 'Thoracic kyphosis: Range in normal subjects.' *Am J Roentgenol 134*, 979–983.

Fox, A., Wanivenhaus, F. and Rodeo, S. (2012) 'The basic science of the patella: Structure, composition, and function.' *J Knee Surg 25*, 2, 127–141.

Fredrickson, B., Baker, D., McHolick, W., Yuan, H. and Lubicky, J. (1984) 'The natural history of spondylolysis and spondylolisthesis.' *J Bone Joint Surg Am 66*, 5, 699–707.

Freke, M., Kemp, J., Svege, I., Risberg, M., Semciw, A. and Crossley, K. (2016) 'Physical impairments in symptomatic femoroacetabular impingement: A systematic review of the evidence.' *Br J Sports Med 50*, 1180.

Fryar, C., Chen, T.-C. and Li, X. (2012) *Prevalence of Uncontrolled Risk Factors for Cardiovascular Disease: United States, 1999–2010.* Hyattsville, MD: National Center for Health Statistics. Accessed on 17/06/2020 at www.cdc.gov/nchs/data/databriefs/db103.pdf.

Frymann, V. (1971) 'A study of the rhythmic motions of the living cranium.' *J Am Osteopath Assoc 70*, 9, 928–945.

Gaeta, M., Minutoli, F., Vinci, S., Salamone, I. *et al.* (2006) 'High-resolution CT grading of tibial stress reactions in distance runners.' *American Journal of Roentgenology 187*, 3, 789–793.

Ganapathy, A., Sadeesh, T. and Rao, S. (2015) 'Morphometric analysis of foot in young adult individuals.' *World Journal of Pharmacy and Pharmaceutical Sciences 4*, 8, 980–993.

Ganz, R., Parvizi, J., Beck, M., Leunig, M., Nötzli, H. and Siebenrock, K. (2003) 'Femoroacetabular impingement: A cause for osteoarthritis of the hip.' *Clin Orthop Relat Res 417*, 112–120.

García Díez, A., Tomás Batlló, X., Pomés Talló, J. and Amo Conill, M. (2009) 'Sacroiliac joints: Osteoarthritis or arthritis.' *Reumatol Clin 5*, 1, 40–43.

Garrett, W. (1996) 'Muscle strain injuries.' *Am J Sports Med 24*, S2–S8.

Gavish, I. and Brenner, B. (2011) 'Air travel and the risk of thromboembolism.' *Intern Emerg Med 6*, 2, 113–116.

GBD 2017 Disease and Injury Incidence and Prevalence Collaborators (2018) 'Global, regional, and national incidence, prevalence, and years lived with disability for 354 diseases and injuries for 195 countries and territories, 1990–2017: A systematic analysis for the Global Burden of Disease Study 2017.' *The Lancet 392*, 10159, 1789–1858.

Geisser, M., Haig, A., Wallbom, A. and Wiggert, E. (2004) 'Pain related fear, lumbar flexion, and dynamic EMG among persons with chronic musculoskeletal low back pain.' *Clin J Pain 20*, 61–69.

Gillies, H. and Chalmers, J. (1970) 'The management of fresh ruptures of the tendo achillis.' *J Bone Joint Surg Am 52*, 337–343.

Giuriato, G., Pedrinolla, A., Schena, F. and Venturelli, M. (2018) 'Muscle cramps: A comparison of the two-leading hypothesis.' *Journal of Electromyography and Kinesiology 41*, 89–95.

Glass, R., Norton, K., Mitre, S. and Kang, E. (2002) 'Pediatric ribs: A spectrum of abnormalities.' *Radiographics 22*, 1, 87–104.

Gollehon, D., Torzilli, P. and Warren, R. (1987) 'The role of the posterolateral and cruciate ligaments in the stability of the human knee: A biomechanical study.' *J. Bone Jt. Surg 69*, 233–242.

Gray, H., Standring, S., Ellis, H. and Berkovitz, B. (2005) *Gray's Anatomy: The Anatomical Basis of Clinical Practice, 39th ed.* New York: Elsevier Churchill Livingtone.

Greendale, G., Huang, M., Karlamangla, A., Seeger, L. and Crawford, S. (2009) 'Yoga decreases kyphosis in senior women and men with adult-onset hyperkyphosis: Results of a randomized controlled trial.' *J Am Geriatrics Society 57*, 9, 1569–1579.

Greenhalgh, T. (2000) *How to Read a Paper: The Basics of Evidence Based Medicine.* London: BMJ.

Gregg, E., Sorlie, P., Paulose-Ram, R., Gu, Q. *et al.* (2004) 'Prevalence of lower-extremity disease in the US adult population >=40 years of age with and without diabetes: 1999–2000 national health and nutrition examination survey.' *Diabetes Care 27*, 1591–1597.

Griffin, R., Dickenson, E., O'Donnell, J., Agricola, R. *et al.* (2016) 'The Warwick Agreement on femoroacetabular impingement syndrome (FAI syndrome): An international consensus statement.' *British Journal of Sports Medicine 50*, 1169–1176.

Groh, M. and Herrera, J. (2009) 'A comprehensive review of hip labral tears.' *Curr Rev Musculoskelet Med 2*, 105–117.

Gross, A., Kay, T., Paquin, J., Blanchette, S. *et al.* (2015) 'Exercises for mechanical neck disorders.' Cochrane Database of Systematic Reviews, 1.

Gross, K., Felson, D., Niu, J., Hunter, D. *et al.* (2011) 'Association of flat feet with knee pain and cartilage damage in older adults.' *Arthritis Care Res 63*, 937–944.

Grover, R. and Rakhra, K. (2010) 'Pes anserine bursitis: An extra-articular manifestation of gout.' *Bulletin of the NYU Hospital for Joint Diseases 68*, 1, 46–50.

Guanche, C. and Sikka, R. (2005) 'Acetabular labral tears with underlying chondromalacia: A possible association with high-level running.' *Arthroscopy 21*, 5, 580–585.

Gubler, D., Mannion, A., Schenk, P., Gorelick, M. *et al.* (2010) 'Ultrasound tissue Doppler imaging reveals no delay in abdominal muscle feed-forward activity during rapid arm movements in patients with chronic low back pain.' *Spine 35*, 1506–1513.

Hagins, M., States, R., Selfe, T. and Innes, K. (2013) 'Effectiveness of yoga for hypertension: Systematic review and meta-analysis.' *Evidence-Based Complementary and Alternative Medicine 2013.*

Hallin, R. (1983) 'Sciatic pain and the piriformis muscle.' *Postgrad Med 74*, 69–72.

Handa, V., Pannu, H., Siddique, S., Gutman, R., VanRooyen, J. and Cundiff, G. (2003) 'Architectural differences in the bony pelvis of women with and without pelvic floor disorders.' *Obstet Gynecol 102*, 1283–1290.

Hannan, T., Felson, D. and Pincus, T. (2000) 'Analysis of the discordance between radiographic changes and knee pain in osteoarthritis of the knee.' *J Rheumatol 27*, 1513–1517.

Hanson, E., Mishra, R., Chang, D., Perkins, T. *et al.* (2010) 'Sagittal whole-spine magnetic resonance imaging in 750 consecutive outpatients: Accurate determination of the number of lumbar vertebral bodies, Clinical article, Journal of Neurosurgery.' *Spine 12*, 47–55.

Harvard Medical School (2007) *National Comorbidity Survey (NCS)*. Accessed on 17/06/2020 at www.hcp.med.harvard.edu/ncs/index.php.

Heron, M. (2019) 'Deaths: Leading causes for 2017.' *National Vital Statistics Reports 68*, 6.

Hill, M. (2019) *Embryology Musculoskeletal System – Bone Development Timeline*. UNSW Embryology. Accessed on 17/06/2020 at https://embryology.med.unsw.edu.au/embryology/index.php/Musculoskeletal_System_-_Bone_Development_Timeline.

Hirschmann, M. and Müller, W. (2015) 'Complex function of the knee joint: The current understanding of the knee.' *Knee Surg Sports Traumatol Arthrosc 23*, 2780.

Hogg-Johnson, S., van der Velde, G., Carroll, L., Holm, L. *et al.* (2008) 'The burden and determinants of neck pain in the general population: Results of the Bone and Joint Decade 2000–2010 Task Force on Neck Pain and Its Associated Disorders.' *Spine 33*, S39–S51.

Howell, E. (2012) 'Pregnancy-related symphysis pubis dysfunction management and postpartum rehabilitation: Two case reports.' *Journal of the Canadian Chiropractic Assoc 56*, 2, 102–111.

Huang, J. and Zager, E. (2004) 'Thoracic outlet syndrome.' *Neurosurgery 55*, 897–903.

Hunt, D., Clohisy, J. and Prather, H. (2007) 'Acetabular tears of the hip in women.' *Phys Med Rehabil Clin N Am 18*, 3, 497–520.

Hunter, D., Niu, J., Felson, D., Harvey, W. *et al.* (2007) 'Knee alignment does not predict incident osteoarthritis: The Framingham osteoarthritis study.' *Arthritis & Rheumatism 56*, 1212–1218.

Ibrahim, I., Khan, W., Goddard, N. and Smitham, P. (2012) 'Carpal tunnel syndrome: A review of the recent literature.' *The Open Orthopaedics Journal 6*, suppl 1, 69–76.

Ingraham, S. (2003) 'The role of flexibility in injury prevention and athletic performance: Have we stretched the truth?' *Minnesota Medicine 86*, 5, 58–61.

Ingvarsson, T. (2000) 'Prevalence and inheritance of hip osteoarthritis in Iceland.' *Acta Orthop Scand Suppl 298*, 1–46.

Insall, J., Falvo, K. and Wise, D. (1976) 'Chondromalacia Patellae: A prospective study.' *J Bone Joint Surg Am 58*, 1, 1–8.

Iyer, S. and Kim, H. (2016) 'Cervical radiculopathy.' *Curr Rev Musculoskelet Med 9*, 272–280.

Jackson, R., Simmons, E. and Stripinis, D. (1983) 'Incidence and severity of back pain in adult idiopathic scoliosis.' *Spine 8*, 7, 749–756.

Jacob, H. and Kissling, R. (1995) 'The mobility of the sacroiliac joints in healthy volunteers between 20 and 50 years of age.' *Clin Biomech 10*, 352–361.

Jankovic, D., Peng, P. and van Zundert, A. (2013) 'Brief review. Piriformis syndrome: Etiology, diagnosis, and management.' *J Can Anesth 60*, 1003–1012.

Jarvik, J., Hollingworth, W., Heagerty, P., Haynor, D., Boyko, E. and Deyo, R. (2005) 'Three-year incidence of low back pain in an initially asymptomatic cohort: Clinical and imaging risk factors.' *Spine 30*, 1541–1548.

Jobe, F. and Ciccotti, M. (1994) 'Lateral and medial epicondylitis of the elbow.' *J American Academy of Orthopaedic Surgeons 2*, 1, 1–8.

Johnson, V. and Hunter, D. (2014) 'The epidemiology of osteoarthritis.' *Best Pract Res Clin Rheumatol 28*, 5–15.

Johnston, R., Cahalan, R., Bonnett, L., Maguire, M. *et al.* (2019) 'General health complaints and sleep associated with new injury within an endurance sporting population: A prospective study.' *Journal of Science and Medicine in Sport 23*, 3, 252–257.

Jung, D., Koh, E. and Kwon, O. (2011) 'Effect of foot orthoses and short-foot exercise on the cross-sectional area of the abductor hallucis muscle in subjects with pes planus: A randomized controlled trial.' *J Back Musculoskelet Rehabil 24*, 4, 225–231.

Kalen, V. and Brecher, A. (1988) 'Relationship between adolescent bunions and flatfeet.' *Foot Ankle 8*, 6, 331–336.

Kalichman, L., Kim, D., Li, L., Guermazi, A., Berkin, V. and Hunter, D. (2009) 'Spondylolysis and spondylolisthesis: Prevalence and association with low back pain in the adult community-based population.' *Spine 34*, 2, 199–205.

Kamkar, A., Irrgang, J. and Whitney, S. (1993) 'Nonoperative management of secondary shoulder impingement syndrome.' *J Orthop Sports Phys Ther 17*, 212–224.

Kapandji, I. (2010) *The Physiology of the Joints, 6th ed.* London: Churchill Livingstone.

Karadimas, E., Trypsiannis, G. and Giannoudis, P. (2011) 'Surgical treatment of coccygodynia: An analytic review of the literature.' *Eur Spine J 20*, 5, 698–705.

Katz, J. and Harris, M. (2008) 'Lumbar spinal stenosis.' *N Engl J Med 358*, 818–825.

Kavaja, L., Lähdeoja, T., Malmivaara, A. and Paavola, M. (2018) 'Treatment after traumatic shoulder dislocation: A systematic review with a network meta-analysis.' *British Journal of Sports Medicine 52*, 1498–1506.

Kavounoudias, A., Roll, R. and Roll, J. (2001) 'Foot sole and ankle muscle inputs contribute jointly to human erect posture regulation.' *J Physiol 532*, 869–878.

Keenan, C. and White, R. (2007) 'The effects of race/ethnicity and sex on the risk of venous thromboembolism.' *Curr Opin Pulm Med 13*, 5, 377–383.

Kegel, A. (1948) 'Progressive resistance exercise in the functional restoration of the perineal muscles.' *Am J Obstet Gynecol 56*, 238–249.

Kelsey, J., Githens, P., Walter, S., Southwick, W. *et al.* (1984) 'An epidemiological study of acute prolapsed cervical intervertebral disc.' *J Bone Joint Surg Am 66*, 907–914.

Kendall, F., McCreary, E., Province, P., Rodgers, M. and Romanin, W. (2005) *Muscle Testing and Function with Posture and Pain, 5th ed.* Philadelphia, PA: Lippincott Williams & Wilkins.

Kerry, R., Bennett, M., Bibby, S., Kester, R. and Alexander, R. (1987) 'The spring in the arch of the human foot.' *Nature 325*, 147–149.

Ketola, S., Lehtinen, J. and Arnala, I. (2017) 'Arthroscopic decompression not recommended in the treatment of rotator cuff tendinopathy: A final review of a randomised controlled trial at a minimum follow-up of ten years.' *Bone Joint J 99*, 6, 799–805.

Khushboo, D., Amrit, K. and Mahesh, M. (2014) 'Correlation between diastasis rectus abdominis and lumbopelvic pain and dysfunction.' *Indian J Physiother Occup Ther 8*, 210–214.

Kibsgårda, T., Røisea, O., Sturesson, B., Röhrl, S. and Stuge, B. (2014) 'Radiosteriometric analysis of movement in the sacroiliac joint during a single-leg stance in patients with long-lasting pelvic girdle pain.' *Clinical Biomechanics 29*, 4, 406–411.

Kim, D., Kim, C. and Son, S. (2018) 'Neck pain in adults with forward head posture: Effects of craniovertebral angle and cervical range of motion.' *Osong Public Health and Research Perspectives 9*, 6, 309–313.

Kim, M., Yi, C., Weon, J., Cynn, H., Jung, D. and Kwon, Y. (2015) 'Effect of toe-spread-out exercise on hallux valgus angle and cross-sectional area of abductor hallucis muscle in subjects with hallux valgus.' *Journal of Physical Therapy Science 27*, 4, 1019–1022.

Kinkade, S. (2007) 'Evaluation and treatment of acute low back pain.' *Am Fam Physician 75*, 8, 1181–1188.

Korkala, O., Gronblad, M., Liese, P. and Karaharju, E. (1985) 'Immunohistochemical demonstration of nociceptors in the ligamentous structures of the lumbar spine.' *Spine 10*, 156–157.

Koroulakis, A. and Agarwal, M. (2019) 'Anatomy, Head and Neck, Lymph Nodes.' In *StatPearls*. Treasure Island, FL: StatPearls Publishing. Accessed on 17/06/2020 at www.ncbi.nlm.nih.gov/books/NBK513317.

Koseki, T., Kakizaki, F., Hayashi, S., Nishida, N. and Itoh, M. (2019) 'Effect of forward head posture on thoracic shape and respiratory function.' *J Phys Ther Sci 31*, 63–68.

Koski, K., Luukinen, H., Laippala, P. and Kivela, S. (1996) 'Physiological factors and medications as predictors of injurious falls by elderly people: A prospective population-based study.' *Age Ageing 25*, 29–38.

Kosuge, D., Yamada, N., Azegami, S., Achan, P. and Ramachandran, M. (2013) 'Management of developmental dysplasia of the hip in young adults.' *The Bone & Joint Journal 95*, B6, 732–737.

Krabak, B., Laskowski, E., Smith, J., Stuart, M. and Wong, G. (2001) 'Neurophysiologic influences on hamstring flexibility: A pilot study.' *Clinical Journal of Sport Medicine 11*, 4, 241–246.

Kravtsov, P., Katorkin, S., Volkovoy, V. and Sizonenko, Y. (2016) 'The influence of the training of the muscular component of the musculo-venous pump in the lower extremities on the clinical course of varicose vein disease.' *Vopr Kurortol Fizioter Lech Fiz Kult 93*, 6, 33–36.

Le, H., Lee, S., Nazarian, A. and Rodriguez, K. (2017) 'Adhesive capsulitis of the shoulder: Review of pathophysiology and current clinical treatments.' *Shoulder and Elbow 9*, 2, 75–84.

Lee, M., Cassinelli, E. and Riew, D. (2007) 'Prevalence of cervical spine stenosis: Anatomic study in cadavers.' *Journal Bone and Joint Surgery 89*, 2, 376–380.

Lee, M., Perez-Rossello, J. and Weissman, B. (2009) 'Pediatric developmental and chronic traumatic conditions, the osteochondroses, and childhood osteoporosis.' In B. Weissman (ed.) *Imaging of Arthritis and Metabolic Bone Disease.* Philadelphia, PA: Saunders Elsevier.

Lee, T., Chay, S. and Kim, H. (2016) 'Diagnosis of flatfoot deformity.' *J Korean Foot Ankle Soc 20*, 1, 1–5.

Levangie, P. and Norkin, C. (2005) *Joint Structure and Function: A Comprehensive Analysis, 4th ed.* Philadelphia, PA: The F.A. Davis Company.

Levin, D., Nazarian, L., Miller, T., O'Kane, P. *et al.* (2005) 'Lateral epicondylitis of the elbow: US findings.' *Radiology 237*, 1, 230–234.

Levinger, P., Menz, H., Fotoohabadi, M., Feller, J., Bartlett, J. and Bergman, N. (2010) 'Foot posture in people with medial compartment knee osteoarthritis.' *J Foot Ankle Res 3*, 29–36.

Lewis, C. and Sahrmann, S. (2006) 'Acetabular labral tears.' *Physical Therapy 86*, 1, 110–121.

Lewis, J. (2011) 'Subacromial impingement syndrome: A musculoskeletal condition or a clinical illusion?' *Physical Therapy Reviews 16*, 5, 388–398.

Liaw, L., Hsu, M., Liao, C., Liu, M. and Hsu, A. (2011) 'The relationships between inter-recti distance measured by ultrasound imaging and abdominal muscle function in postpartum women: A 6-month follow-up study.' *J Orthop Sports Phys Ther 41*, 435–443.

Lievense, A., Bierma-Zeinstra, S., Schouten, B., Bohnen, A., Verhaar, J. and Koes, B. (2005) 'Prognosis of trochanteric pain in primary care.' *Br J Gen Pract 55*, 199–204.

Liow, R., McNicholas, M., Keating, J. and Nutton, R. (2003) 'Ligament repair and reconstruction in traumatic dislocation of the knee.' *Bone and Joint Journal 85*, 845–851.

Littlewood, C., May, S. and Walters, S. (2013) 'Epidemiology of rotator cuff tendinopathy: A systematic review.' *Shoulder Elbow 5*, 256–265.

Loudon, J., Goist, H. and Loudon, K. (1998) 'Genu recurvatum syndrome.' *J Orthop Sports Phys Ther 27*, 5, 361–367.

Loukas, M., Louis, R., Wartmann, C., Shane Tubbs, R. *et al.* (2008) 'An anatomic investigation of the serratus posterior superior and serratus posterior inferior muscles.' *Surg Radiol Anat 30*, 119–123.

Lu, Y., Rosner, B., Chang, G. and Fishman, L. (2016) 'Twelve-minute daily yoga regimen reverses osteoporotic bone loss.' *Top Geriatr Rehabil 32*, 2, 81–87.

Lynn, S., Padilla, R. and Tsang, K. (2012) 'Differences in static- and dynamic-balance task performance after 4 weeks of intrinsic-foot-muscle training: The short-foot exercise versus the towel-curl exercise.' *Journal of Sport Rehabilitation 21*, 327–333.

MacDermid, J. and Doherty, T. (2004) 'Clinical and electrodiagnostic testing of carpal tunnel syndrome: A narrative review.' *J Orthop Sports Phys Ther 34*, 10, 565–588.

Maffulli, N. (1999) 'Rupture of the Achilles tendon.' *J Bone Joint Surg Am 81*, 1019–1036.

Maffulli, N., Wong, J. and Almekinders, L. (2003) 'Types and epidemiology of tendinopathy.' *Clin Sports Med 22*, 675–692.

Majewski, M., Susanne, H. and Klaus, S. (2006) 'Epidemiology of athletic knee injuries: A 10-year study.' *The Knee 13*, 3, 184–188.

Malvankar, S. and Khan, W. (2011) 'Evolution of the Achilles tendon: The athlete's Achilles heel?' *Foot 21*, 4, 193–197.

Mannion, A., Caporaso, F., Pulkovski, N. and Sprott, H. (2012) 'Spine stabilisation exercises in the treatment of chronic low back pain: A good clinical outcome is not associated with improved abdominal muscle function.' *Eur Spine J 21*, 1301–1310.

Manske, R. and Prohaska, D. (2008) 'Diagnosis and management of adhesive capsulitis.' *Curr Rev Musculoskelet Med 1*, 180–189.

Masharawi, Y., Rothschild, B., Dar, G., Peleg, S. *et al.* (2004) 'Facet orientation in the thoracolumbar spine: Three-dimensional anatomic and biomechanical analysis.' *Spine 29*, 16, 1755–1763.

McCaffrey, R. and Park, J. (2012) 'The benefits of yoga for musculoskeletal disorders: A systematic review of the literature.' *J Yoga Phys Ther 2*, 5, 1–11.

McCarthy, J., Noble, P., Schuck, M., Wright, J. and Lee, J. (2001) 'The Otto E Aufranc Award: The role of labral lesions to development of early degenerative hip disease.' *Clin Orthop 393*, 25–37.

McCoy, G., McCrea, J., Beverland, D., Kernohan, G. and Mollan, R. (1987) 'Vibration arthrography as a diagnostic aid in diseases of the knee.' *J Bone Joint Surg (Br) 69-B*, 2, 288–293.

McHugh, M. and Cosgrave, C. (2010) 'To stretch or not to stretch: The role of stretching in injury prevention and performance.' *Scand J Med Sci Sports 20*, 169–181.

McInnes, I. and Schett, G. (2011) 'The pathogenesis of rheumatoid arthritis.' *N Engl J Med 365*, 2205–2219.

McKenzie, J. (1955) 'The foot as a half-dome.' *Br Med J 1*, 1068–1069.

Menz, B. and Lord, S. (2001) 'The contribution of foot problems to mobility impairment and falls in community-dwelling older people.' *J Am Geriatr Soc 49*, 1651–1656.

Menz, B. and Lord, S. (2005) 'Gait instability in older people with hallux valgus.' *Foot Ankle 26*, 483–489.

Millar, A. (1979) 'Strains of the posterior calf musculature ("tennis leg").' *Am J Sports Med 7*, 3, 172–174.

Misuri, G., Colagrande, S., Gorini, M., Iandelli, I. *et al.* (1997) 'In vivo ultrasound assessment of respiratory function of abdominal muscles in normal subjects.' *Eur Respir J 10*, 12, 2861–2867.

Mitchell, F. and Pruzzo, N. (1971) 'Investigation of voluntary and primary respiratory mechanisms.' *J Am Osteopath Assoc 70*, 10, 1109–1113.

Moen, M., Tol, J., Weir, A., Steunebrink, M. and De Winter, T. (2009) 'Medial tibial stress syndrome: A critical review.' *Sports Med 39*, 7, 523–546.

Moore, K. (ed.) (1992) *Clinically Oriented Anatomy, 3rd ed.* Baltimore, MD: Williams and Wilkins.

Morgan, P., LaPrade, R., Wentorf, F., Cook, J. and Bianco, A. (2010) 'The role of the oblique popliteal ligament and other structures in preventing knee hyperextension.' *Am J Sports Med 38*, 550–557.

Morrey, B. (ed.) (2000) *The Elbow and its Disorders.* Philadelphia, PA: WB Saunders.

Moseley, J., O'Malley, K., Petersen, N., Menke, T. *et al.* (2002) 'A controlled trial of arthroscopic surgery for osteoarthritis of the knee.' *N Engl J Med 347*, 81–88.

Mow, V., Fithian, D. and Kelly, M. (1989) 'Fundamentals of Articular Cartilage and Meniscus Bio-mechanics.' In J. Ewing (ed.) *Articular Cartilage and Knee Joint Function: Basic Science and Arthroscopy.* New York: Raven Press.

Mueller, W. (1982) *The Knee: Form, Function, and Ligament Reconstruction.* New York: Springer.

Neer, C. (1972) 'Anterior acromioplasty for the chronic impingement syndrome in the shoulder: A preliminary report.' *J Bone Joint Surg Am 54*, 41–50.

Neer, C. (1983) 'Impingement lesions.' *Clin Orthop Relat Res 173*, 70–77.

Neumann, D. (2009) *Kinesiology of the Musculoskeletal System: Foundations for Physical Rehabilitation, 2nd ed.* St. Louis, MO: Mosby.

Neviaser, A. and Neviaser, R. (2011) 'Adhesive capsulitis of the shoulder.' *J Am Acad Orthop Surg 19*, 536–542.

Nix, S., Smith, M. and Vicenzino, B. (2010) 'Prevalence of hallux valgus in the general population: A systematic review and metaanalysis.' *J Foot Ankle Res 3*, 21.

Nordenvall, R., Bahmanyar, S., Adami, J., Stenros, C., Wredmark, T. and Felländer-Tsai, L. (2012) 'A population-based nationwide study of cruciate ligament injury in Sweden, 2001–2009: Incidence, treatment, and sex differences.' *Am J Sports Med 40*, 1808–1813.

Norton, B., Sahrmann, S. and Van Dillen, L. (2004) 'Differences in measurements of lumbar curvature related to gender and low back pain.' *J Orthop Sports Phys Ther 34*, 9, 524–534.

O'Donnell, J., Devitt, B. and Arora, M. (2018) 'The role of the ligamentum teres in the adult hip: Redundant or relevant? A review.' *Journal of Hip Preservation Surgery 5*, 1, 15–22.

Ohshima, H., Hirano, N., Osada, R., Matsui, H. and Tsuji, H. (1993) 'Morphologic variation of lumbar posterior longitudinal ligament and the modality of disc herniation.' *Spine 18*, 16, 2408–2411.

Øiestad, B., Engebretsen, L., Storheim, K. and Risberg, M. (2009) 'Knee osteoarthritis after anterior cruciate ligament injury: A systematic review.' *Am J Sports Med 37*, 1434–1443.

Oikonomou, A. and Prassopoulos, P. (2011) 'CT imaging of blunt chest trauma.' *Insights Imaging 2*, 3, 281–295.

Oschman, J., Chevalier, G. and Brown, R. (2015) 'The effects of grounding (earthing) on inflammation, the immune response, wound healing, and prevention and treatment of chronic inflammatory and autoimmune diseases.' *Journal of Inflammation Research 8*, 83–96.

Outerbridge, R. and Outerbridge, H. (2001) 'The etiology of chondromalacia patellae.' *Clinical Orthopaedics and Related Research 389*, 5–8.

Padua, L., Coraci, D., Erra, C., Pazzaglia, C. *et al.* (2016) 'Carpal tunnel syndrome: Clinical features, diagnosis, and management.' *Lancet 15*, 12, 1273–1284.

Paine, R. and Voight, M. (2013) 'The role of the scapula.' *International Journal of Sports Physical Therapy 8*, 5, 617–629.

Palazzo, C., Nguyen, C., Lefevre-Colau, M., Rannou, F. and Poiraudeau, S. (2016) 'Risk factors and burden of osteoarthritis.' *Annals of Physical and Rehabilitation Medicine 59*, 3, 134–138.

Palmgren, T., Grönblad, M., Virri, J., Kääpä, E. and Karaharju, E. (1999) 'An immunohistochemical study of nerve structures in the annulus fibrosus of human normal lumbar intervertebral discs.' *Spine 24*, 2075–2079.

Palsson, T., Gibson, W., Darlow, B., Bunzli, S. *et al.* (2019) 'Changing the narrative in diagnosis and management of pain in the sacroiliac joint area.' *Physical Therapy 99*, 11, 1511–1519.

Parvizi, J., Bican, O., Bender, B., Mortazavi, S. *et al.* (2009) 'Arthroscopy for labral tears in patients with developmental dysplasia of the hip: A cautionary note.' *The Journal of Arthroplasty 24*, 6, suppl 1.

Pascoe, M. and Bauer, I. (2015) 'A systematic review of randomized control trials on the effects of yoga on stress measures and mood.' *Journal of Psychiatric Research 68*, 270–282.

Pattyn, E., Verdonk, P., Steyaert, A., Vanden Bossche, L. *et al.* (2001) 'Vastus medialis obliquus atrophy: Does it exist in patellofemoral pain syndrome?' *Am J Sports Med 39*, 1450–1455.

Peat, M. (1986) 'Functional anatomy of the shoulder complex.' *Phys Ther 66*, 1855–1865.

Peelle, M., Della Rocca, G., Maloney, W., Curry, M. and Clohisy, J. (2005) 'Acetabular and femoral radiographic abnormalities associated with labral tears.' *Clin Orthop Relat Res 441*, 327–333.

Penning, L. (2000) 'Psoas muscle and lumbar spine stability: A concept uniting existing controversies. Critical review and hypothesis.' *Eur Spine J 9*, 577–585.

Perkins, B., Olaleye, D. and Bril, V. (2002) 'Carpal tunnel syndrome in patients with diabetic polyneuropathy.' *Diabetes Care 25*, 3, 565–569.

Petersen, J. and Hölmich, P. (2005) 'Evidence based prevention of hamstring injuries in sport.' *British Journal of Sports Medicine 39*, 319–323.

Phalen, G. (1966) 'The carpal-tunnel syndrome.' *J Bone and Joint Surg Am 48*, 380–383.

Picerno, V., Ferro, F., Adinolfi, A., Valentini, E., Tani, C. and Alunno, A. (2015) 'One year in review: The pathogenesis of rheumatoid arthritis.' *Clin Exp Rheumatol 33*, 551–558.

Planès, S., Villier, C. and Mallaret, M. (2016) 'The nocebo effect of drugs.' *Pharmacology Research & Perspectives 4*, 2.

Polatin, P., Kinney, R., Gatchel, R., Lillo, E. and Mayer, T. (1993) 'Psychiatric illness and chronic low-back pain. The mind and spine: Which goes first?' *Spine 18*, 66–71.

Polly, D., Kilkelly, F., McHale, K., Asplund, L., Mulligan, M. and Chang, A. (1996) 'Measurement of lumbar lordosis: Evaluation of intraobserver, interobserver, and technique variability.' *Spine 21*, 13, 1530–1535.

Posadzki, P. and Ernst, E. (2011) 'Yoga for asthma? A systematic review of randomized clinical trials.' *Journal of Asthma 48*, 6, 632–639.

Puddu, G., Ippolito, E. and Postacchini, F. (1976) 'A classification of Achilles tendon disease.' *Am J Sports Med 4*, 145–150.

Qiu, J. and Kang, J. (2017) 'Exercise associated muscle cramps – a current perspective.' *Scientific Pages Sports Med 1*, 1, 3–14.

Radhakrishnan, K., Litchy, W., O'Fallon, W. and Kurland, L. (1994) 'Epidemiology of cervical radiculopathy: A population-based study from Rochester, Minnesota, 1976 through 1990.' *Brain 117*, 325–335.

Raizada, V. and Mittal, R. (2008) 'Pelvic floor anatomy and applied physiology.' *Gastroenterology Clinics of North America 37*, 3, 493–509.

Ralston, S. (2013) 'Paget's disease of bone.' *Atlas Genet Cytogenet Oncol Haematol 17*, 10, 726–727.

Rao, B. and Joseph, B. (1992) 'The influence of footwear on the prevalence of flat foot: A survey of 2300 children.' *The Journal of Bone and Joint Surgery 74-B*, 4, 525–527.

Rathleff, M., Mølgaard, C., Fredberg, U., Kaalund, S. *et al.* (2015) 'HL strength training and plantar fasciopathy.' *Scand J Med Sci Sports 25*, 292–300.

Renstrom, F. and Lynch, S. (1999) 'Acute injuries of the ankle.' *Foot Ankle Clin 4*, 697–711.

Richardson, C., Snijders, C., Hides, J., Damen, L., Pas, M. and Storm, J. (2002) 'The relation between the transversus abdominis muscles, sacroiliac joint mechanics, and low back pain.' *Spine 27*, 4, 399–405.

Riddle, D. and Schappert, S. (2004) 'Volume of ambulatory care visits and patterns of care for patients diagnosed with plantar fasciopathy: A national study of medical doctors.' *Foot Ankle Int 25*, 303–310.

Ridola, C. and Palma, A. (2001) 'Functional anatomy and imaging of the foot.' *Ital J Anat Embryol 106*, 85–98.

Rixe, J., Glick, J., Brady, J. and Olympia, R. (2013) 'A review of the management of patellofemoral pain syndrome.' *Phys Sportsmed 41*, 19–28.

Robbins, S. and Hanna, A. (1987) 'Running-related injury prevention through barefoot adaptations.' *Med Sci Sports Exerc 19*, 2, 148–156.

Roberts, S., Evans, H., Trivedi, J. and Menage, J. (2006) 'History and pathology of the human intervertebral disc.' *J Bone Joint Surg Am 88*, suppl 2, 10–14.

Robertson, C. (2010) 'Joint crepitus – are we failing our patients?' *Physiother Res Int 15*, 185–188.

Robertson, C., Hurley, M. and Jones, F. (2017) 'People's beliefs about the meaning of crepitus in patellofemoral pain and the impact of these beliefs on their behaviour: A qualitative study.' *Musculoskelet Sci Pract 28*, 59–64.

Rubin, D. (2007) 'Epidemiology and risk factors for spine pain.' *Neurol Clin 25*, 2, 353–371.

Ruch, W. (1997) *Atlas of Common Subluxations of the Human Spine and Pelvis.* Boca Raton, FL: CRC Press.

Sambandam, S., Khanna, V., Gul, A. and Mounasamy, V. (2015) 'Rotator cuff tears: An evidence-based approach.' *World J Orthop 6*, 11, 902–918.

Sanders, R., Hammond, S. and Rao, N. (2007) 'Diagnosis of thoracic outlet syndrome.' *J Vascular Surgery 46*, 3, 601–604.

Saraceni, N., Kent, P., Ng, L., Campbell, A., Straker, L. and O'Sullivan, P. (2019) 'To flex or not to flex? Is there a relationship between lumbar spine flexion during lifting and low back pain? A systematic review with meta-analysis.' *J Orthop Sports Phys Ther 50*, 3, 121–130.

Sathyaprabha, T., Murthy, H. and Murthy, B. (2001) 'Efficacy of naturopathy and yoga in bronchial asthma: A self-controlled matched scientific study.' *Indian J Physiol Pharmacol 45*, 80–86.

Schneider, D., von Mühlen, D., Barrett-Connor, E. and Sartoris, D. (2004) 'Kyphosis does not equal vertebral fractures: The Rancho Bernardo study.' *J Rheumatol 31*, 4, 747–752.

Schwellnus, M., Derman, E. and Noakes, T. (1997) 'Aetiology of skeletal muscle "cramps" during exercise: A novel hypothesis.' *J Sports Sci 15*, 277–285.

Seres, J. (2003) 'Evaluating the complex chronic pain patient.' *Neurosurg Clin N Am 14*, 339–352.

Sharma, M. and Haider, T. (2013a) 'Yoga as an alternative and complementary treatment for patients with low back pain: A systematic review.' *J Evidence-Based Comp & Alter Med 18*, 1, 23–28.

Sharma, M. and Haider, T. (2013b) 'Yoga as an alternative and complementary therapy for patients suffering from anxiety: A systematic review.' *J Evidence-Based Comp & Alter Med 18*, 1, 15–22.

Shaw, J., Sicree, R. and Zimmet, P. (2010) 'Global estimates of the prevalence of diabetes for 2010 and 2030.' *Diabetes Res Clin Pract 87*, 4–14.

Sheikhhoseini, R., Shahrbanian, S., Sayyadi, P. and O'Sullivan, K. (2018) 'Effectiveness of therapeutic exercise on forward head posture: A systematic review and meta-analysis.' *J Manipulative and Physiological Therapeutics 41*, 6, 530–539.

Sheridan, M. and Hannafin, J. (2006) 'Upper extremity: Emphasis on frozen shoulder.' *Orthop Clin North Am 37*, 531–539.

Shiri, R., Viikari-Juntura, E., Varonen, H. and Heliövaara, M. (2006) 'Prevalence and determinants of lateral and medial epicondylitis: A population study.' *American Journal of Epidemiology 164*, 11, 1065–1074.

Siegel, L., Vandenakker-Albanese, C. and Siegel, D. (2012) 'Anterior cruciate ligament injuries: Anatomy, physiology, biomechanics, and management.' *Clin J Sport Med 22*, 349–355.

Silva, J., Chagas, C., Torres, D., Servidio, L., Vilela, A. and Chagas, W. (2010) 'Morphological analysis of the fabella in Brazilians.' *Int J Morphol 28*, 105–110.

Silverstein, M., Heit, J., Mohr, D., Petterson, T., O'Fallon, W. and Melton, L. (1998) 'Trends in the incidence of deep vein thrombosis and pulmonary embolism: A 25-year population-based study.' *Arch Intern Med 158*, 6, 585–593.

Singh, I., Ajita, R. and Singh, N. (2015) 'Variation in the number of sacral pieces.' *IOSR Journal of Dental and Medical Sciences 14*, 2, 106–108.

Singh, R., Kishore, L. and Kaur, N. (2014) 'Diabetic peripheral neuropathy: Current perspective and future directions.' *Pharmacol Res 80*, 21–35.

Slauterbeck, J., Kousa, P., Clifton, B., Naud, S. *et al.* (2009) 'Geographic mapping of meniscus and cartilage lesions associated with anterior cruciate ligament injuries.' *J Bone Joint Surg Am 91*, 2094–2103.

Small, K., McNaughton, L. and Matthews, M. (2008) 'A systematic review into the efficacy of static stretching as part of a warm-up for the prevention of exercise-related injury.' *Research in Sports Medicine 16*, 3, 213–231.

Smallwood Lirette, L., Chaiban, G., Tolba, R. and Eissa, H. (2014) 'Coccydynia: An overview of the anatomy, etiology, and treatment of coccyx pain.' *Ochsner Journal 14*, 1, 84–87.

Smith, C., Kruger, M., Smith, R. and Myburgh, K. (2008) 'The inflammatory response to skeletal muscle injury.' *Sports Med 38*, 947–969.

Smith, C., Vacek, P., Johnson, R., Slauterbeck, J. *et al.* (2012) 'Risk factors for anterior cruciate ligament injury: A review of the literature – part 1: neuromuscular and anatomic risk.' *Sports Health 4*, 1, 69–78.

Snook, S., Webster, B., McGorry, R., Fogleman, M. and McCann, K. (1998) 'The reduction of chronic nonspecific low back pain through the control of early morning lumbar flexion: A randomized controlled trial.' *Spine 23*, 23, 2601–2607.

Spitznagle, T., Leon, F. and Dillen, L. (2007) 'Prevalence of diastasis recti abdominals in uro-gynecological population.' *Int Urogynecol J Pelvic Floor Dysfunct 18*, 321–328.

Steinke, H., Hammer, N., Slowik, V., Stadler, J. *et al.* (2010) 'Novel insights into the sacroiliac joint ligaments.' *Spine 35*, 3, 257–263.

Stocker, B., Nyland, J., Caborn, D., Sternes, R. and Ray, J. (1997) 'Results of the Kentucky high school football knee injury survey.' *J Ky Med Assoc 95*, 11, 458–464.

Sung, K. and Yu, I. (2014) 'Acquired adult flatfoot: Pathophysiology, diagnosis, and nonoperative treatment.' *J Korean Foot Ankle Soc 18*, 3, 87–92.

Symmons, D., Turner, G., Webb, R., Asten, P. *et al.* (2002) 'The prevalence of rheumatoid arthritis in the United Kingdom: New estimates for a new century.' *Rheumatology 41*, 7, 793–800.

Talasz, H., Kremser, C., Kofler, M., Kalchschmid, E. *et al.* (2011) 'Phase-locked parallel movement of diaphragm and pelvic floor during breathing and coughing – a dynamic MRI investigation in healthy females.' *Int Urogynecol J 22*, 1, 61–68.

Tatu, L., Parratte, B., Vuillier, F., Diop, M. and Monnier, G. (2001) 'Descriptive anatomy of the femoral portion of the iliopsoas muscle: Anatomical basis of anterior snapping of the hip.' *Surg Radiol Anat 23*, 6, 371–374.

Taunton, J., Ryan, M., Clement, D., McKenzie, D., Lloyd-Smith, D. and Zumbo, B. (2002) 'A retrospective case-control analysis of 2002 running injuries.' *Br J Sports Med 36*, 95–101.

Tetsworth, K. and Paley, D. (1994) 'Malalignment and degenerative arthropathy.' *Orthop Clin North Am 25*, 367–377.

Teunis, T., Lubberts, B., Reilly, B. and Ring, D. (2014) 'A systematic review and pooled analysis of the prevalence of rotator cuff disease with increasing age.' *Journal of Shoulder and Elbow Surgery 23*, 12, 1913–1921.

Thomee, R., Augustsson, J. and Karlsson, J. (1999) 'Patellofemoral pain syndrome: A review of current issues.' *Sports Med 28*, 245–262.

Toohey, A., LaSalle, T., Martinez, S. and Polisson, R. (1990) 'Iliopsoas bursitis: Clinical features, radiographic findings, and disease associations.' *Semin Arthritis Rheum 20*, 41–47.

Torry, M., Schenker, M., Martin, H., Hogoboom, D. and Philippon, M. (2006) 'Neuromuscular hip biomechanics and pathology in the athlete.' *Clin Sports Med 25*, 179–197.

Tresch, F., Dietrich, T., Pfirrmann, C. and Sutter, R. (2017) 'Hip MRI: Prevalence of articular cartilage defects and labral tears in asymptomatic volunteers. A comparison with a matched population of patients with femoroacetabular impingement.' *J. Magn. Reson. Imaging 46*, 440–451.

Trobisch, P., Suess, O. and Schwab, F. (2010) 'Idiopathic scoliosis.' *Deutsches Arzteblatt International 107*, 49, 875–884.

Trojian, T. and Tucker, A. (2019) 'Plantar fasciopathy.' *Am Fam Physician 99*, 12, 744–750.

Uchiyama, S., Itsubo, T., Nakamura, K., Kat, H., Yasutomi, T. and Momose, T. (2010) 'Current concepts of carpal tunnel syndrome: Pathophysiology, treatment, and evaluation.' *J Orthop Sci 15*, 1–13.

Ukoha, U., Egwer, O., Okafov, I., Ogugua, C. and Igwenagu, N. (2012) 'Pes planus: Incidence in adult population in Anambra state, Southeast Nigeria.' *Indian Journal of Basic and Applied Medical Research 3*, 3, 166–168.

Umlauf, D., Frank, S., Pap, T. and Bertrand, J. (2010) 'Cartilage biology, pathology, and repair.' *Cellular and Molecular Life Sciences 67*, 4197–4211.

US Department of Health and Human Services (2004) *Bone Health and Osteoporosis: A Report of the Surgeon General.* Rockville, MD: DoHHS.

van Middelkoop, M., Kolkman, J., van Ochten, J., Bierma-Zeinstra, S. and Koes, B. (2007) 'Course and predicting factors of lower-extremity injuries after running a marathon.' *Clin J Sport Med 17*, 1, 25–30.

van Staa, T., Selby, P., Leufkens, H., Lyles, K., Sprafka, J. and Cooper, C. (2002) 'Incidence and natural history of Paget's disease of bone in England and Wales.' *J Bone Miner Res 17*, 465–471.

van Tulder, M., Becker, A., Bekkering, T., Breen, A. *et al.* (2006) 'European guidelines for the management of acute nonspecific low back pain in primary care.' *Eur Spine J 15*, suppl 2, S169–S191.

Vasseljen, O., Woodhouse, A., Bjørngaard, J. and Leivseth, L. (2013) 'Natural course of acute neck and low back pain in the general population: The HUNT study.' *Pain 154*, 8, 1237–1244.

Vleeming, A., Schuenke, M., Masi, A., Carreiro, J., Danneels, L. and Willard, F. (2012) 'The sacroiliac joint: An overview of its anatomy, function and potential clinical implications.' *J Anat 221*, 537–567.

Voight, M. and Thomson, B. (2000) 'The role of the scapula in the rehabilitation of shoulder injuries.' *J Athl Training 35*, 3, 364–372.

Weppler, C. and Magnusson, P. (2010) 'Increasing muscle extensibility: A matter of increasing length or modifying sensation?' *Physical Therapy 90*, 3, 438–449.

Wertli, M., Rasmussen-Barr, E., Weiser, S., Bachmann, L. and Brunner, F. (2014) 'The role of fear avoidance beliefs as a prognostic factor for outcome in patients with nonspecific low back pain: A systematic review.' *Spine 14*, 5, 816–836.

Wheatley, W., Krome, J. and Martin, D. (1996) 'Rehabilitation programmes following arthroscopic meniscectomy in athletes.' *Sports Med 21*, 447–456.

Wieland, L., Skoetz, N., Pilkington, K., Vempati, R., D'Adamo, C. and Berman, B. (2017) 'Yoga treatment for chronic non-specific low back pain.' *Cochrane Database of Systematic Reviews 1*.

Wiese, C., Keil, D., Rasmussen, A. and Olesen, R. (2019) 'Injury in yoga asana practice: Assessment of the risks.' *J Bodyw Mov Ther 23*, 3, 479–488.

Wiewelhove, T., Döweling, A., Schneider, C., Hottenrott, L. *et al.* (2019) 'A meta-analysis of the effects of foam rolling on performance and recovery.' *Front Physiol 10*, 376.

Wijdicks, C., Griffith, C., Johansen, S., Engebretsen, L. and LaPrade, R. (2010) 'Injuries to the medial collateral ligament and associated medial structures of the knee.' *J Bone Joint Surg Am 92*, 5, 1266–1280.

Wilke, H., Wolf, S., Claes, L., Arand, M. and Wiesend, A. (1995) 'Stability of the lumbar spine with different muscle groups.' *Spine 20*, 192–198.

Wiltse, L. and Winter, R. (1983) 'Terminology and measurement of spondylolisthesis.' *J Bone Joint Surg Am 65*, 768–772.

Wong, J., Côté, P., Quesnele, J., Stern, P. and Mior, S. (2014) 'The course and prognostic factors of symptomatic cervical disc herniation with radiculopathy: A systematic review of the literature.' *The Spine Journal 14*, 1781–1789.

Wong, Y. (2007) 'Influence of the abductor hallucis muscle on the medial arch of the foot: A kinematic and anatomical cadaver study.' *Foot Ankle Int 28*, 5, 617–620.

Woon, J., Perumal, V., Maigne, J. and Stringer, M. (2013) 'CT morphology and morphometry of the normal adult coccyx.' *Eur Spine J 22*, 4, 863–870.

World Health Organization (2012) *Depression: A Global Crisis.* Accessed on 08/09/2021 at https://www.who.int/mental_health/management/depression/wfmh_paper_depression_wmhd_2012.pdf?Ua=1.

Xu, G., Liu, B., Sun, Y., Du, Y. *et al.* (2018) 'Prevalence of diagnosed type 1 and type 2 diabetes among US adults in 2016 and 2017: Population-based study.' *BMJ 362*, k1497.

Yamamoto, A., Takagishi, K., Osawa, T. and Yanagawa, T. (2010) 'Prevalence and risk factors of a rotator cuff tear in the general population.' *Journal of Shoulder and Elbow Surgery 19*, 1, 116–120.

Yan, Y., Li, Q., Wu, C., Pan, X. *et al.* (2018) 'Rate of presence of 11 thoracic vertebrae and 6 lumbar vertebrae in asymptomatic Chinese adult volunteers.' *J Orthop Surg Res 13*, 124.

Yang, J., Tibbetts, A., Covassin, T., Cheng, G., Nayar, S. and Heiden, E. (2012) 'Epidemiology of over-use and acute injuries among competitive collegiate athletes.' *Journal of Athletic Training 47*, 2, 198–204.

Yang, N., Chen, H., Phan, D., Yu, I.-L. *et al.* (2011) 'Epidemiological survey of orthopedic joint dislocations based on nationwide insurance data in Taiwan, 2000–2005.' *BMC Musculoskelet Disord 12*, 253.

Yates, B. and White, S. (2004) 'The incidence and risk factors in the development of medial tibial stress syndrome among naval recruits.' *Am J Sports Med 32*, 3, 772–780.

Yoga Journal and Yoga Alliance (2016) *The 2016 Yoga in America Study.* Accessed on 17/06/2020 at www.yogaalliance.org/Portals/0/2016%20Yoga%20in%20America%20Study%20RESULTS.pdf.

Zeng, C., Xiong, J., Wang, J.C., Inoue, H. *et al.* (2016) 'The evaluation and observation of "hidden" hypertrophy of cervical ligamentum flavum, cervical canal, and related factors using kinetic magnetic resonance imaging.' *Global Spine Journal 6*, 2, 155–163.

Zeng, S., Dong, X., Dang, R., Wu, G. *et al.* (2012) 'Anatomic study of fabella and its surrounding structures in a Chinese population.' *Surg Radiol Anat 34*, 65–71.

FURTHER READING
AND RESOURCES

Accessible Yoga: Poses and
Practices for Every Body
Jivana Heyman 2019
Shambhala Publications, Boulder
ISBN: 978 1 61180 712 7

The Ehlers-Danlos Society
www.ehlers-danlos.com

Reconciling Biomechanics with
Pain Science
www.greglehman.ca/
pain-science-workbooks

Hypermobility on the Yoga Mat:
A Guide to Hypermobility-Aware
Yoga Teaching and Practice
Jess Glenny 2021
Singing Dragon, London
ISBN: 978 1 78775 465 2

PainScience.com
www.painscience.com

Yoga Biomechanics: Stretching Redefined
Jules Mitchell 2019
Handspring Publishing, Fountainhall
ISBN: 978 1 90914 161 2

Yoga for Depression: A Compassionate
Guide to Relieve Suffering Through Yoga
Amy Weintraub 2004
Broadway Books, New York
ISBN: 978 0 76791 450 5

Yoga Therapy for Arthritis
Dr Steffany Moonaz and Erin Byron 2018
Singing Dragon, London
ISBN: 978 0 85701 302 6

Your Body, Your Yoga
Bernie Clark 2016
Wild Strawberry Productions, Vancouver
ISBN: 978 0 96876 653 8

SUBJECT INDEX

AUTHOR INDEX